EMBRACING THE WOUNDS OF POST-TRAUMATIC STRESS DISORDER

An Invitation to Heal

EMBRACING THE WOUNDS OF POST-TRAUMATIC STRESS DISORDER

An Invitation to Heal

Bernadette Cioch

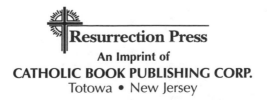

Resurrection Press
An Imprint of
CATHOLIC BOOK PUBLISHING CORP.
Totowa • New Jersey

First published in April, 2008 by
Catholic Book Publishing/Resurrection Press
77 West End Road
Totowa, NJ 07512

ISBN 978-1-933066-10-3

Library of Congress Catalog Card Number: 2007940984

Cover design by Geoffrey Butz

Printed in the United States of America

1 2 3 4 5 6 7 8 9

www.catholicbookpublishing.com

This book is dedicated to the memory
of those who lost their lives in the crash of TWA Flight 800
and
to their families and to the rescuers who responded
and suffered as a result of their selfless commitment
to helping others.

If we believe those who have died are free,
let us who remain also believe that their wish for us
is to live out our lives in freedom.

The ultimate purpose of this book is to give witness to the love of God, the mercy of the Son of God, Jesus Christ, and the healing power of the Holy Spirit. With faith and trust in Jesus, all human beings can overcome their trials by seeking God's grace of acceptance and unconditional love. I believe that sharing my story of Post-Traumatic Stress Disorder can be a source of understanding, guidance, insight, healing and hope for all those who walk this road with us, those who live with us, and those who treat us.

Since PTSD affects memory and concentration this book is written in short chapters and understandable language so the reader may not be overwhelmed by its content.

Contents

Acknowledgments

"Whether he tries to enter into a dislocated world, relate to a convulsive generation, or speak to a dying man, his service will not be perceived as authentic unless it comes from a heart wounded by the suffering about which he speaks."   Henri J.M. Nouwen, *The Wounded Healer*

TO the God of my creation, without your unconditional love I could not have embarked upon such a painful journey which in turn gave me the great gift of being a <u>wounded healer</u>. Thank you also for the abundant joy that comes from being able to relate through this book to others who know the pain of PTSD. By sharing it may they also know the hope. To God goes the glory.

To my husband Joseph, my children and grandchildren, you are truly the wind beneath my wings. I will always be grateful for all of the support, love, light and joy that you bring into my life.

To John Bowman, Ph.D., a psychologist of pure skill, endless patience, deep compassion, bright spirit and a much needed sense of humor. Thank you for sharing my brokenness and my hope.

To my friend Dean Calloway for countless hours of editing and typing. Thank you for the encouraging words you always had for me and your sensitivity to others who are hurting. I am grateful for doing all of this on your own time and with no other reward than a simple Thank You.

To my beautiful friends Annette and Ed Echart, founders of Bridge for Peace ministry. You always had faith in me and my story. Your belief in the healing power of the Holy Spirit led you to be my greatest strength dur-

ing my years of healing and writing. Your spiritual guidance will be with me always. Peace of Jesus be with you
always.

To my spiritual director Josephine Daspro, CSJ, D.Min.
who prayerfully companioned me to understand my relationship to God through some very dark hours and also
to the mystical understanding that comes with suffering.
Thank you for helping me to know that through it all,
God is.

To Rev. Robert McGuire, SJ, who helped me to trust the
knowledge and wisdom I had through the gifts of the
Holy Spirit to go forward as wounded healer and continue to live out God's purpose for my life. Thank you for
believing in me even when I didn't believe in myself.

To my friend Terry Shirreffs who from the beginning of
writing my story encouraged me to let others touch my
wounds. My sincerest thank you.

To Emilie Cerar and Donna Rogers Kranich for your
editing suggestions. I took courage and grew from your
honesty and love. Thank you for caring.

Foreword

IN the spring of 1990 I was appointed District Psychologist for the Setauket Fire District on Long Island and immediately began to conduct Stress Management Workshops for fire department and emergency medical services personnel. In the course of these meetings and discussions, it became apparent that coping with highly traumatic events would require more than the application of relaxation exercises and cognitive behavior techniques. It was in pursuit of these additional tools that I first met Bernadette Cioch. I recall her open invitation to meet with her and her supervisor at her office to review a program for conducting Critical Incident Stress Management (CISM) for firefighters and emergency medical personnel throughout Suffolk County. I could not help but be impressed with her boundless enthusiasm and heartfelt commitment to "helping the helper." This was the phrase she used to describe the countywide initiative to provide psychological help to all volunteer fire and emergency services departments that requested it by sending a team of trained personnel to conduct structured debriefings to help defuse the debilitating impact of exposure to highly traumatic events. There was no way of knowing then that seven years later I would be called upon to help this particular helper in her painful journey back from the trauma of TWA Flight 800 to her renewed life as a beacon for healing and hope once again.

By inviting us to join her in the depths of her experience through Post-Traumatic Stress Disorder, we were able to observe firsthand what clinicians have come to know. The impact of psychological trauma is pervasive through the totality of the human organism. The Jesuit scholar Pierre Teilhard de Chardin observed that, "We are not human beings having a spiritual experience. We are spiritual beings having a human experience." Bernadette's story is a testimony to her belief in herself as a spiritual being above all else. In the face of the reconstruction of all her ways of organizing herself, others, and life itself, she was able to demonstrate how faith and hope are the guideposts to healing from trauma in the presence of God's eternal love.

If you have the courage to act in your own behalf and join Bernadette in her journey through this book, then you too will be blessed by this belief.

John J. Bowman, Ph.D.

Introduction

CIVILIAN or rescuer, every human person has a threshold. The human psyche has limits. No one knows when an event will be so painful and will cause strong emotional and physical aftershocks that are too powerful for them to handle themselves.

All people, in every walk of life, have stress. Stress is caused by your job, family and social life. Yet emergency services related occupations have their own unique brand of stressors and, yes, they are often worse than those experienced in other careers.

Most people do not see in a lifetime what emergency service personnel can encounter in one day. Unlike other "regular" 9-to-5 jobs, emergency service work makes demands on time, energy, ability and/or emotions. It piles multiple stressors high on an individual's plate—strictly regulated, highly intense training, multiple restrictions on practice, constant changes in workplace and schedule, as well as low pay and no pay for volunteers. Added to these, often there is little recognition or support from administration. Worse yet, police, fire, military and emergency medical personnel handle the most tragic and violent situations: the aftereffects of child abuse, combative patients, suicide, murder, severe injuries and gory fatalities in car crashes and fires, large-scale disasters incorporating mass loss of human life and the deaths of colleagues in the line of duty.

In the field of emergency services, high burnout rates are also associated with high rates of attrition. The loss of trained personnel has been reported to be as high as 40 percent after two to five years of employment (McSwain

NE, Skelton MB: "Burnout-real or imagined?" *Emergency Care Quarterly,* 1980). According to an article by Steven R. Hawks and Ronald L. Hammond (*Journal of Emergency Medical Services Communications,* September 1990, p. 50), the presence of identical external stressors can produce different stress responses in an individual based on the unique mental perception of the stressor. This is because burnout and high turnover are not only caused by job-related stress but by external factors including one's personal life, as well as fitness levels, education and training, stress management and support.

Over the past 15 years, several studies have significantly improved our understanding of the problem. Field personnel are trained regularly to recognize the causes, signs and symptoms and to effectively manage stress. Time is set aside for Critical Incident Stress Defusings and Debriefings (CISD) which are frequently used during and after acute stress and traumatic events. In direct contrast, emergency services personnel set high standards for themselves and often have the unspoken conviction that they need to keep their problems private. They are people who want to succeed and who are trained to succeed. It is often difficult for them to share their feelings. Yet, even though they may be the strongest of people, a seasoned veteran must face the fact that people die despite the best efforts of the rescuer.

This is the real and inspiring story of one such person who built a very successful career within the emergency medical service system over the course of 27 years. In 1971 Bernadette Cioch started as an emergency medical technician and later as an advanced critical care tech. As the founder and first chief of an advanced life support volunteer ambulance corps, she was an active riding member of the ambulance corps for 23 years. During five years of this time she flew trauma medi-vacs.

In 1982 Bernadette was hired by the Suffolk County Department of Health, Division of Emergency Medical Services to coordinate the advanced life support training program for all of the County's fire and EMS personnel. Two years later in 1984, she initiated the Suffolk County Critical Incident Stress Management Team to give psychological and emotional assistance to rescuers and civilians at the scene of a traumatic incident and to follow up with a formal debriefing that emphasizes ventilation of feelings, emotions and other reactions. The team is composed of peer support counselors such as police officers, EMS personnel and firefighters along with mental health professionals. Bernadette was the director, instructor, team leader and peer counselor for over 13 years.

Working together with colleagues and legislators, laws were set in place that changed the course of emergency services funding regulations in New York and paved the way for the stress management module in the New York State emergency medical technician course curriculum. She was a maverick who lobbied tirelessly for passage of progressive governmental policy.

Although this is a story of a person who made a positive—often life saving—difference in the lives of thousands of patients and colleagues, it is ironically a story of injury and loss, denial and depression into the spiraling, out-of-control terror and debilitation associated with PTSD, set off by the trauma of one of the biggest airline disasters within U.S. borders.

This story is not just for emergency service workers. It is for all those who suffer with PTSD–the woman who is raped in the workplace, the battered spouse, the abused child, the survivor of a motor vehicle crash, the person left alone by the sudden death of a loved one, the soldier returning home from war or those affected by the horrors of the World Trade Center disaster and other acts of terrorism across the globe. On some level we are all survivors of the tragic events of 9/11, but it is estimated that hundreds of thousands of people in New York City alone are still feeling the effects of that dark day in our nation's history. How do we help the person who cannot get back on the subway to get to work? How do we help the person who gets up in the morning and cannot function past making a cup of coffee? Or the person who sees no purpose in going on? How do we help these people and all those who love and minister to them?

It is the intention of this author to educate and give hope, to bring light into the darkness, to bring PTSD out of the shadows and to dispel the stigma of shame and render it powerless in the presence of a living, protective, merciful and all-mighty God.

Donna Rogers Kranich

1

A Traumatic Encounter:
The Flight 800 Air Disaster

The woods are lovely, dark and deep,
But I have promises to keep,
And miles to go before I sleep,
And miles to go before I sleep.

—Robert Frost

JULY 17, 1996, started out like any other day. I was vacationing at Montauk Point—a very serene waterfront resort town at the eastern end of Long Island, New York. Around 5 a.m. I took a long walk along an empty and quiet beach listening to the sounds of the seagulls and the waves rolling to shore. I love the ocean; it is always a source of relaxation and peace for me. As I watched the fishing boats go out to sea, I sat in the sand and took a deep breath of the clean ocean air. All the turmoil of my life just seemed to fade away. Later I walked down the beach and up the street to the church of St. Theresa the Little Flower where I attended Mass and sat for a long time before the Blessed Sacrament. Today more than ever I would need His presence very close to me.

The rest of the day was uneventful until 8:40 that evening when a breaking news flash came across the television screen: A TWA 747 JET LINER WENT DOWN OFF THE COAST OF LONG ISLAND. My heart started pounding as a million thoughts ran through my mind. Was it Suffolk County? Were there survivors? If not, what were the imprints of horror that I would be faced with in the next few hours? Was the Critical Incident Stress Management Team going to be needed?

One phone call to Chief of Operations at the dispatch center for Fire Rescue and Emergency Services told the story. My fears were confirmed: a TWA 747 carrying 230 passengers had crashed off of Suffolk County at Center Moriches. As the director of the CISM Team, I went into immediate action. There was a need and as a rescuer I responded. That is what a rescuer does. Period.

The trip from Montauk Point to my office in Yaphank where the team would meet was a one-hour trip. This gave me a little time to collect my thoughts and form a preliminary plan. One hour from serenity to insanity. That hour was probably the longest hour of my life. I knew the first order of business was to pray for the victims, the families, the rescuers and myself. I trusted the Lord knew what was in my heart and I said the Our Father. Knowing it would be bad, I prayed for His help through this dark night. I left the rest in God's hands and began to coordinate a plan for the team who had already assembled at the dispatch center in Yaphank. They were a beautiful sight. They also knew we were going to visit hell that night and yet they all showed up. True professionals, yet all volunteers. This is what we were trained for, and now, all of our background experience in emergency services brought us to this time and place. We were ready.

At 11 p.m. the call came in from the Suffolk County Police Department to respond to the scene. I found out quickly that my division director was already at the scene but could not be reached. My two immediate supervisors were in Albany and would not be back until the following day. This left me feeling very alone and unsupported. Now I had to make more decisions beyond directing the CISM team which was a tremendous responsibility in itself.

Some of these decisions included getting coverage for the emergency operations center in Yaphank. This center is where all county emergency response agencies gather to work together in a disaster situation. Our division of emergency medical services needed to be represented. In the absence of any other command personnel at the EMS office, I dispatched two of our division employees to respond and rotate twelve-hour shifts, and I directed Fire Rescue dispatch to relay all non-disaster and routine calls to the Nassau County CISM team until further notice.

Suffolk County has in place a civilian CISM team. This team takes care of the families of the victims. My team takes care of the rescuers. It was not yet clear whether the families were coming out to Long Island or if they were going to stay in New York City. However, the civilian team director was out of the country and I could not reach his backup. Now I was really concerned about my team and the stress was mounting. We were not prepared to deal with civilians and this put us on overload very quickly. Just then the phone rang and it was the sergeant in charge of the police marine bureau requesting team members to respond to his personnel. I gave him the number of the police department CISM team. We had trained their team just a few weeks prior so now they could take care of their own personnel. I next tried to reach the Nassau County team director for additional backup, but he was not available.

It was time for us to respond to the Coast Guard station in Center Moriches where body recovery was already in progress. Every person on my team was highly trained, and I had every confidence in them. However, despite our many years of experience, we had never been required to provide the intense service which Flight 800 would require. There was no turning back. The first responding team members led by assistant team director John Fleishmann went to the scene immediately. I followed with additional team members when they arrived.

As we approached Atlantic Avenue off Main Street in Center Moriches, which was a fifteen minute ride from the dispatch center in Yaphank, we met our first police checkpoint. Emotions were running high as we would have to pass through twelve more police checkpoints before reaching the Coast Guard station which took another fifteen minutes to complete. We had proper identification and knew the importance of the screening process. Terrorism was a consideration because no one knew what brought this plane down. All I knew was that there was an explosion. To make a government feel vulnerable, terrorists like to target rescuers, so safety was a real concern. The last stretch of the ride brought the Coast Guard station into view. It was an eerie sight because I knew just on the other side of that building a nightmare was unfolding. We passed by the media who were crowding the street and had squeezed through the fence where security cut them off. Every major news station was represented.

Upon arrival at the scene I was informed that it was a recovery mission and there was little hope for survivors. I felt terribly empty and sad as I wondered what happened to this plane. I felt intense compassion for the victims and relatives. I just couldn't imagine losing someone I loved in such a horrible way.

Disaster scenes present a somewhat carnival atmosphere and this was no exception. Many agencies literally set up camp. Tents rise, busses and trucks bringing in food and supplies seem to be everywhere. Police, fire and emergency medical services respond to the area. Coast Guard command personnel, Red Cross, FBI, NTSB, AT&T phone communication operations, and National Guard moved in a dizzying array of uniforms.

Meanwhile, I was unable to respond to numerous messages from Fire Rescue dispatch from various agencies, because within hours of the crash, cellular phone service became nonexistent. This failure of a much needed communications system was created by the press locking out all available cell sites which created a highly frustrating and unsafe situation. At this crucial time I was completely cut off not only from returning messages but also from soliciting additional help.

As we approached the back dock of the Coast Guard station I was trying to prepare myself for the worst. I didn't realize it then, but there was nothing to prepare me for what I was about to encounter. I had been in emergency medical services for twenty-six years, but I had never experienced anything of this magnitude. The recovery process was well in progress. Boat after boat just kept bringing in dead and broken bodies of the victims—men, women and children. The scene was surreal. These were people who only hours ago were living out their lives not knowing the horrible tragedy that would befall them. I thought to myself, "They never knew what was coming."

At the same time, I felt some kind of change take place in my body. It was very uncomfortable. I knew I was emotionally and physically injured. From what I knew of the critical incident stress reaction I immediately questioned, "Was this it?" I felt sick to my stomach, totally overwhelmed and then everything went into slow motion. This lasted for what seemed like an eternity, but it was only seconds that passed. I knew I had a job to do and I was determined to do it. I picked up my cell phone which I knew was not working. I pretended to be making a phone call so I could clear my head and deal with my emotions in a constructive way.

Very quickly I began to feel some real anger. Where are You God? Where were You? How could You have let this happen? I need to see You here and I need to see You here NOW. Just then I looked down on the lower dock and saw a Rabbi praying the Psalms. Because of my very strong faith, I was comforted just knowing that someone was praying for the victims and for us. It gave me the grace to continue.

The Coast Guard officers requested that we work with their personnel as they were coming off the boats. We worked all through the night and well into the next day doing defusings and one-on-one peer counseling for over five hundred people. I can remember the pain of one young Coast Guard woman who said, " You know before tonight I never saw a dead person." She just sat there staring out into the darkness. It was the THOUSAND MILE STARE—that long stare with a blank look in one's eyes totally disbelieving of what just occurred. By five that evening it would be me in that same thousand mile stare.

By approximately 2 a.m. many bodies had been recovered but there were still no body bags on site. One of the boats brought in the body of an unclothed young woman and a young Coast Guard officer found a blanket and covered her. His mother would have been proud of him. As a mother, the pain of seeing so many dead children went to the core of my soul. There were so many children on this plane who had died far too early in their young lives. One mother was still holding her child—they fell thirteen thousand feet and she never let go of her child.

They kept coming in. Children, backpacks, luggage, parts of the plane, the pilot's hat and then a teddy bear. The teddy bear got to everyone. It was the symbol of a child. Whatever else we were able to deny, we could not deny that teddy bear. The death of a child is one of the highest forms of stress a rescuer can face, and we had to face that reality over and over in a very short time span.

Private boaters went out to help find survivors but they found only the dead. There was no one to save. I could see the shock and disbelief they were in. One boat brought in the torso of one of the victims and as the body was being taken off the boat I saw in the shadows the figure of a young child shivering with fear. I don't know why the child was on the boat, but I couldn't help but think about the long term psychological effects this would have on her. I knew at that moment not all the victims of Flight 800 died in the crash. All of the passengers died but not all of the victims. Some would carry the scars for life. We comforted them and gave everyone that we ministered to that night a copy of the Common Signs and Symptoms of Traumatic Stress (see pp. 54-55).

The scene got worse as the night went on—bringing in bodies and body parts hour after hour for what seemed like an eternity. There were shocked and emotionally numb rescuers everywhere. The Red Cross was passing food to them over dead bodies. My thoughts of the victims and their families were intensifying by the minute. I just could not grasp the magnitude of the loss. I felt overwhelmed. I wanted to run away but in my heart I knew I could not leave because that was not who I was as a professional, a person, a rescuer. We were the only support team there and a lot of people needed our help. I was injured but I was going to stay with my team and fellow rescuers. My feelings had to be put on hold. Later I would feel the pain. Later I would cry.

The night hours were bad and the sights we were exposed to were horrible, but nothing was as bad as when the dawn came. The darkest hour was truly dawn. What I tried not to see before was unavoidable. The horror before me was unbearable as I looked across the docks and saw the refrigerator truck. A tractor-trailer full of bodies. The whole scene had the sense of not being real. In high contrast, however, the pain on the faces of the rescuers was very real—contorted and stressed. Their faces told of the imprints of horror that they had to endure all through the night. Their pain was a reflection of my own and it was hard to look at.

In spite of the unforgettable horror of this experience, I will always carry two positive memories with me from that night: the quiet reverence with which every broken human person was handled and the presence of the faithful Rabbi who prayed there all night. As the day progressed body recovery slowed down as the number of body bags multiplied. The helicopters never stopped. In and out all night and day. There was always someone who had to get to the scene or leave the scene. Walking around the side of the Coast Guard station in the open field, I saw what looked like a sea of luggage. There were hundreds of suitcases, carry ons, backpacks, etc. The passengers had been carrying so much stuff—things they would no longer need. I thought about everything I carry around with me every day. I longed for a simpler place and time. I thought about the people who died and how they had such hope and joy about their trip to Paris. My mother and I had taken that same flight only three years prior on our visit to Lourdes. It could have been us.

I had been on the go now for a very long time and I was exhausted, overwhelmed, in shock and in deep grief. I walked over to a table and sat down. It was now about six in the evening—about 22 hours since the plane went down. There were a lot of mental health counselors and CISM teams there now so I could relax a little. I was glad that they did not have to endure the events of the previous hours. The worst part of the recovery mission was over, but my job was not yet over.

I called the team together and released them from the scene. We had to be debriefed within forty-eight hours. I walked back to the dock and found myself staring out at the sea looking at a rainbow that had formed in the sky. I thought about the contrast of good and evil, the plane crash and the rainbow—the biblical sign of God's covenant with His people. I was grateful for God's presence in the calming beauty of that rainbow. I was even more grateful that I could still feel His presence. That was His grace for me at that moment.

∞ FOR REFLECTION ∞

"The Rabbi Prayed"

Looking out at the sea
The memory unwelcome but yet to be
A warm July night
A doomed flight
God sent us to care
God help us to bear
And the Rabbi prayed.

Death all around
No life to be found
All joined together
In a monumental endeavor
To bring home the lost
To their families at all cost
And the Rabbi prayed.

Many hours had passed
No relief at last
Backpacks and teddy bears
God please dry our tears
Parents without children
Children without parents
And the Rabbi prayed.

Tons of twisted steel
The scene was surreal
Rescuers downhearted
For those now departed
And the Rabbi prayed.

As time goes by
Less and less we cry
Yet deep in our souls
We are changed forever.

Lord thank you for the rainbow
Which lifted hearts that were low
And for letting the dark night give way
To the light of a new day.
We will heal with your love
For this I pray.

෯෯෯෯ ෯෯෯෯

If I rise on the wings of the dawn
and settle at the farthest limits of the sea,
even there your hand will guide me,
and your right hand will hold me fast.

Psalms 139: 9-10

∞ AN INVITATION TO HEAL ∞

HOW about you? Have you told your story? Is there a safe person whom you can trust with your pain, feelings and emotions—such as a family member, a friend, a therapist, a minister or a spiritual director? When sharing your story, timing is important—it does not have to be done all at once. The ability to face and feel the pain will come over time and in tolerable doses.

Why is it good to talk about our trauma? When we talk about our pain, we feel less alone and it gives others permission to do the same. It gives us the empowerment to move from victim to survivor. It is an experience of being freed not unlike Lazarus being unbound and set free. " I am telling the story; therefore, I have survived. " Owning our survival is an important part of the healing process.

To put the events into words helps transform the memories and emotions associated with the trauma. Telling our story helps us accept some of what we have lost and helps us to integrate the lost parts of ourselves with the new emerging parts that are more connected to reality. It allows us to look forward to who we are now and how we are challenged to heal. We can explore the whole event and its potential for our own personal growth. In this potential lies the possibility of discovering the difference between simply acknowledging the presence of God, and finding a true healing connection to Him.

Questions for Reflection

1. Are you able to sit and talk with Jesus and tell him how alone and isolated you feel?

2. Can you bring all of yourself to the relationship? Even the anger?

3. Do you believe that God as loving Father understands your anguish?

4. What remains real in the ruins of your shattered beliefs? What have you lost? What have you gained? Try to name them.

5. Can you accept the joy you feel as you rediscover parts of you that you thought were gone forever?

6. Has this experience in your life challenged you to grow spiritually? In what way?

2

In Their Memory

For this God is our God for ever and ever; he will be our guide even to the end. Psalms 48:14

MY family was waiting for me when I got home. They were concerned for me and, I guess, suspected I would need to talk. The truth is I could not even begin to tell them what I had just been through. I had no words to describe it. It was just too big. What they saw on TV and what I witnessed at the scene were not even close. I spoke with my family briefly and went to bed. I was too tired too pray. I did manage to sleep that night but was up early to meet with a few team members. We returned to the site and continued our services for a week. During this week we assisted many agencies with crisis intervention and acted as liaisons directing people to the appropriate agencies for the specific help they required. Phone calls—on my cell, in the command post, at work or at home—did not stop for two weeks straight.

Four days later at our Critical Incident Stress Management Team debriefing, it was clear that this disaster had profound effects. All of us were subjected to the

horror of a major mass casualty incident. We were wit-
nesses to the same horror as the people we were there to
help and it took a toll on all of us.

The debriefing took place in my home. I wanted everyone to feel comfortable, so I welcomed them into a safe
place to share their feelings. Most team members were
able to share on a feelings level which helped me to share
some of my own feelings. I found I was more emotional
than usual and this both scared and embarrassed me. I
did not like the feeling of not being in control. I just kept
telling myself this was a normal reaction to an abnormal
event. I knew intellectually that to show my feelings was
ok and very healthy. Yet I did not want to appear "not" ok.
I was still in denial and I needed to be because my work
was not finished.

On Sunday, all responders who wished to participate,
were blessed by the music ministry and priest from a
nearby parish who came to say Mass for us in a tent at the
scene of the crash. It was especially emotional when we
sang "Be Not Afraid." The beautiful and tender vibrations
of the guitar strings touched the strings of my heart as did
the words of the Lord: "I go before you always." In the
depths of my soul I knew he went before all who died in
this plane crash. I trust he took them to his heart before
they suffered any pain. In his love they abide.

On July 24, exactly one week after the crash, a memorial service was held at Smith Point Park in Mastic Beach,
which was just a few miles west of the crash site. The
chairs were set up on the beach facing the water in the
direction the plane went down. It was a beautiful sunny
day. All agencies involved in the rescue and recovery mis-

sion stood side by side forming a corridor for the family members to walk through as they were seated. Each was given a rose to toss into the water as part of the ceremony. A young, pretty woman who had lost her fiancé stopped and kissed each team member and said thank you. I felt the tears well up inside me at her gratitude and love. I looked at the team and every one of them had tears in their eyes. She did us a great service that day. We don't do what we do for the thank you, but when someone says it, it is deeply felt and greatly appreciated.

Then the bagpipers moved into place. They would lead the procession of dignitaries and families through the corridor of rescue personnel to their seats by the water facing the crash site. As they started to play "Amazing Grace" I felt the vibrations go right through me. I could hardly swallow because of the lump in my throat. I knew there were tears falling from my eyes but because we were standing at attention I could not wipe them dry. So I said to myself, "let'em flow." The ceremony was moving and the words were as comforting as they could be. Hundreds of people attended this nondenominational prayer service including George Pataki, the governor of the State of New York and Mayor Rudolph Giuliani. They recalled the dedication and challenging efforts of all the agencies that responded and conveyed a deep sense of gratitude for all of the rescuers' efforts. The main theme for the clergy who spoke was to encourage families and rescuers to, in time, accept what they have experienced and keep the faith. Since the victims of Flight 800 were largely strangers, travelers from 14 nations, it was very moving to hear all of the prayers and love that was shown that day. At the conclusion we walked down to the ocean with the families and threw roses into the water with them. We were able to talk with some of them. They were kind and grateful for our efforts. This was a special time for us all—the beginning of the grief process. I felt empty as if I had nothing left to give. I needed to rest so desperately, but there was still work to be done.

After the memorial I started to arrange formal debriefings. There was very little Fire and EMS involvement because of the nature of the incident so debriefings for them were minimal. The sessions held were primarily for support personnel who were stationed on the docks and were exposed to the emotional trauma of witnessing multiple deaths. One of the most rewarding was the debriefing for the clergy, which was new and very needed. The clergy are a forgotten group that sometimes fall through the cracks. We were assisted by the FBI CISM team peer council member. These Jewish, Protestant and Catholic clergymen were bonded in their service to the dead, and now they were bonded in their need to heal.

I began their debriefing by reading Psalm 21: The Lord My Guardian. After what we had witnessed we were all feeling vulnerable. I trusted by reading the Word of God we would be comforted in remembering the Lord never sleeps. He is with us always even in distress. This was not a normal procedure but then what was normal anymore? While reading the psalm I began to lose ground. I knew I was injured more severely than I had originally thought. I was not ok. My denial was breaking down so I removed myself from the debriefing process until I could consult a mental health provider. It was a decision I made in the moment and it was not an easy one. It hurt to admit to myself and others that I was not ok. I remained faithful to that decision because I knew it was the best thing for me and those whom I was there to serve. Because of all my training I suspected I was dealing with Post-Traumatic Stress.

Three months after the plane crash my work was done. Every "t" was crossed and every "i" was dotted. It was finished. Now I could crash. And I did.

∞ FOR REFLECTION ∞

"The Work Of Angels"

There are times
When words are not enough to say
There are times
When hearts must find another way

When the darkness was more than anyone could bear
You were there, shining everywhere

Like beacons in the night
You lit that lonely place

And, through the mist,
You carried them with silent grace
You could not undo the loss
But you have helped to set them free
Reaching out for them beneath the rolling sea

(chorus)
  We have seen the work of angels
  And it makes a wondrous light
  You have risen from among us

With your wings kept out of sight
You're the finest sons and daughters of America
And you did her proud, because you did it right

And so it's always been
And it will always be
When fate steps in
And life is torn by tragedy

For every heart that's broken,
An angel steps in view
An angel who looks
Very much like you

(repeat chorus)

And when the call goes out again
On some forsaken night
We will hear the sounds of angels taking flight . . .
You're the finest sons and daughters of America . . .

© 1996, P. Petruccelli
Lone Sparrow Music (ASCAP)

∞ AN INVITATION TO HEAL ∞

FOR all people who have lost someone close to them and to all rescuers who have witnessed the death of another human being, I invite you to grieve. This invitation to grieve is an invitation to heal and to heal is to let go and to move forward. Not to forget but to continue with life. How do we find any meaning in a disaster? To have a loved one die in such a sudden and horrible condition is one of the most painful experiences a person will ever have to endure in a lifetime.

Grief is a healthy way to acknowledge loss. It is a necessary process and each has their own timetable for going through the entire process. A supportive atmosphere is essential for a person to navigate this process in a healthy way. Showing pain is not synonymous with weakness—it is actually the opposite. <u>Grieving is a way of releasing very painful feelings and it promotes healing.</u>

When Jesus was told his friend Lazarus had died, he wept. He wept openly. He loved his friend and was experiencing deep sorrow. He was not embarrassed by his outward expression of pain. He used it to move forward and free his friend from the bonds of death just as he continues to free us and our loved ones from the bonds of death. We can be freed from our sorrow but like Jesus we must first feel the feelings and endure the process. This includes rescuers who grieve for people they don't even know.

Some or all of the following support services may be helpful to you.

1. Grief counselors can be of great assistance to help guide and support us gently through this time of confusion, loss and pain. They can also help us see clearly and get our lives back into perspective.
2. Bereavement groups help by providing a sense of family. These groups are a place where we can share our pain and emotions with others who understand. It is also a place to offer each other unconditional love in coping.
3. Critical Incident Stress Debriefing helps to alleviate the feelings of isolation. It helps us explore our pain and share freely in a safe place among our peers. This sharing is a very healing experience. Even when there

are no answers, just the sense of not being alone in this suffering can help us begin to heal.

4. Memorial services and rituals not only honor the dead but are extremely helpful for those left behind. It is comforting to know that our loved one hasn't been forgotten.

After the traumatic crucifixion and death of Jesus, the apostles gathered in the upper room. They were in pain, confused, traumatized and feeling a great loss. In this gathering they shared their pain and fears. They consoled one another. In a sense they were debriefing. Even in this time of suffering we grow and seek new life. The ability to heal and go forward with our lives after a loss is a tribute to us and to the memory of those who have died.

Questions for Reflection

1. Do you believe sharing your feelings is ok? If not, why not?

2. Are you willing to sit with others who are grieving and share your feelings?

3. Will you spend some time in a quiet place with Jesus and allow him to comfort you?

3

The Injury

Cast all your anxiety on him, because he cares about you.
1 Peter 5:7

TEARS. Tears were streaming down my face as I looked around my office. Everything was the same. The pictures, the furniture, the objects on my desk. Everything was the same—except me. I did not know it at the time but I was changed forever.

In 1982 Charles Kurault gave his impressions of the mud slides and deaths that occurred in Santa Cruz, California by stating: "Once you have seen this, something changes inside. Once you have absorbed what nature and the forest can do, once you have seen the majestic glorious redwoods turned into bludgeons and the good earth stirred into soup; once you have seen all this you will never walk the same way in the forest again." Once I saw 230 people die in a major commercial airplane crash; once I saw the broken and dismembered bodies of so many men, women and children; once I saw the pain and suffering of families and rescuers; once I saw all of this I would never be the same again.

Even with all of my training in stress, trauma and coping, because it was me who was injured, in reality I knew very little. I was experiencing the effects of severe trauma. My normal coping mechanisms were not working and I felt like I was losing my mind. I was scared, and I felt truly vulnerable. For me feeling vulnerable and out of control was a fate worse than death. Later, I would come to understand how this place of vulnerability would bring me closer to Jesus. In my fear and need I turned to him for help. He did not fail me.

In the days to come I could not stop asking myself and God: What happened? How did this happen to me? WHY ME? I was always such a strong person. I was the one who took care of everyone else. I was the one people turned to for help. Now I needed help. This was a place I had never been to before and I did not like it one bit. In my anger I started to search for answers I could live with.

I began with what Mr. Webster had to say about trauma. The definition read: "it is a bodily or emotional shock, which often has a lasting psychic effect." I believe that to be true—but incomplete. For me trauma is a deep and painful wounding that devastated my life and affected me on every level of my being.

Trauma has many faces and there are many ways to be injured: living with alcoholism in the family, divorce, rape and sexual abuse of any kind, domestic violence, physical injury, the sudden death of a loved one, witnessing or responding to a mass casualty incident are some of the most prevalent ones. The sudden death of a loved one can be particularly traumatic because the person who goes through this will experience both grief and trauma.

Grief as we know it is a normal biological mechanism that is already in place. Although painful, it is an expected reaction to loss. The body and the emotions will experience the following stages (not necessarily in this order): shock, denial, anger, bargaining, acceptance and reintegration. Most people have had a loss in their lives and can relate to this process. Trauma on the other hand is an extraordinary response with a whole set of signs and symptoms that occur from the unique and individual nature of trauma. A person is having a normal reaction to an abnormal event but it feels unnatural. The traumatized person will ask the same questions I asked. Why can't I get it together? Why can't I concentrate? When will the nightmares go away? So the person who experiences a sudden death loss will experience both grief and trauma symptoms and it is this combination that can overwhelm any person's ability to cope. Most people experience loss and can relate to loss but unless a person has known trauma, they cannot relate to what a traumatized person is going through. This includes therapists who treat trauma survivors, and why it is so important to find experienced counselors.

Sometimes the effects of trauma can be severe and can cause post-traumatic stress disorder. In November of 1996 I was diagnosed with PTSD. I was crushed. I felt guilt and shame. I thought that I brought this on myself. It seemed it must be my fault because of something I did or did not do. The more I learned about PTSD the more I understood that this is not true. PTSD is an anxiety disorder usually accompanied by depression. It has both psychological and physiological components. This injury to the brain is a real medical condition, (see DSM IV for diagnostic criteria). In my heart of hearts I knew it was so even before the diagnosis but I was no less devastated. I had all of the components. I felt the chemical change take place in my body on the dock at the Coast Guard Station. My physical, emotional, mental, social and spiritual well being were not ok and not the same as they were before the injury. My anxiety level was out of control and I was in a deep depression. Memory and concentration became an almost intolerable effort.

It is believed that one out of every thirteen Americans has PTSD on some level. Some people have it and don't know it. Many of our soldiers returning from Iraq are suffering grave symptoms of PTSD and the suicide rates are increasing dramatically. There are those who won't seek help because of the stigma attached to seeing a mental health provider. This is so unfortunate because PTSD can be treated. The difference between a victim and survivor is the victim can't get past the "why me?" They keep trying to be who they were before the trauma. The survivor may visit that place but eventually they reach acceptance and make the decision to move on. The help the Lord sent to me was the willingness to seek the help I needed and the courage to endure the process. I went to places deep within my soul. I went to places of interminable pain.

Those who will not seek help run the risk of using negative coping mechanisms to help ease their pain. Drug and alcohol abuse are at the top of the list. They give immediate relief and are sadly more socially acceptable than seeing a therapist. This is a short fix and in the long run will only make things worse. Social problems can develop because of the symptoms of irritability and the isolation that occurs. By trying to hide the symptoms and keep the feelings locked inside, some people will develop physical problems such as high blood pressure, heart disease, cancer and gastrointestinal problems. Personality changes will cause problems with family and friends—sometimes to the point of divorce and even suicide. Untreated PTSD is dangerous.

Not everyone who experiences trauma will get PTSD but in extreme cases the percentages can reach 25% or more as in the World Trade Center disaster. Eighteen months after the Oklahoma City bombing there was an increase of over 55% at alcohol treatment centers for in patient and out patient care. When these symptoms do appear later it is confusing and very often the connection will not be made that what the person is going through is a result of the original injury. This later manifestation of symptoms is usually caused be a trigger—something similar happens through sight, sound or smell that happened at the time of the event. Traumatic injury can be very complicated and it takes a trained mental health provider to treat it. If you or a loved one is manifesting the effects of a recent or past trauma, it is wise to seek help promptly. Shop wisely.

I will be sharing the details of my treatment more fully in the following chapters.

∽ FOR REFLECTION ∾
Letters from the Soul

Dear Jesus,
As I contemplate your wounds upon the cross I know
they are for love of me. I have wounds, too, but I am
afraid to look at them. Please help me to see within my
wounds the power of your love and mercy. My wounds
show my weakness and my dependence. This is a new
place for me. Only you, O Lord, can save me now. Save
me from this pit of pain and despair. It is dark here, Lord.
It is cold and lonely. Fill this loneliness with your pure
love and restore my health and peace, dear Jesus.

Dear Bernadette,
You are my beloved. Restore your soul I will. Trust in my
ways and in my time. Consider this time with me in the
tomb. We will spend time together. You will learn much
from me here. In my time I will call you out of the tomb
and then you will be raised up on eagles' wings and you
will no longer grow weary. Trust in me, my child.

∽ AN INVITATION TO HEAL ∾

If you have suffered a trauma then you have been deeply hurt. If no one has ever validated your pain then I am validating it now. Why do we need validation? Unless our pain is validated "it is not real." If it is not real, then it can not be resolved. One reason so many people go into delayed stress reaction is because there is no one there to support them. Without support it is difficult to face the truth of what really is. Healing begins when we can face that truth.

Whether your trauma was direct or indirect, intentional or unintentional you have been hurt. If no one has ever said they were sorry to you, then in the name of Jesus I am saying it to you now. When we look to the cross I see Jesus—the ultimate trauma victim. One day when I was contemplating the cross I asked Jesus: Why me? He spoke to my heart and said WHY ME? I never needed to ask him that question again. I know that he has gone before me in all of my suffering. He knows about my pain. He knows I have been to the cross with him and he knows one day I too will come off the cross. When I reflect on his resurrection I feel validated and have great hope for my life. Through the power of the Holy Spirit I know a deep abiding union with my Lord and Savior Jesus Christ. I learned this in the days, weeks, months and even years that followed my trauma. It did not come to me all at once. I learned that the survivor has the key—the willingness to turn their life over to God—and in His infinite wisdom He will lead them to recovery and peace. "Peace, peace to all, both far and near, and I will heal them, says the Lord" (Isa 57:19).

Questions for Reflection

1. What concerns you the most about seeking treatment for PTSD?

2. Can you accept the living God as the center of your support and validation?

3. In the midst of your pain and suffering where do you find God?

4

Losing Ground

"I will lead the blind
and guide them along paths they do not know.
I will turn darkness into light before them
and make straight their winding roads.
These are the things I will do for them,
and I will not forsake them."   Isaiah 42:16

❧

A FTER a traumatic event occurs, society strongly implies, we should go on with our lives as best we can. Keep to a normal routine. Pick up the pieces and move on. This is good advice for those who can do it. However, when I sustained the injury of PTSD, my path was indeed different. I was led in ways that were unfamiliar and I was blind for awhile.

My journal entry on November 18, 1996 (four months after the Flight 800 tragedy) reads: "Today I need to talk about my anger. I realized how angry I was while talking to a friend last night. I was talking about the plane crash and I could feel my whole body tense up. My pulse was racing and I had pain in my chest. I thought I was having a heart attack, but it was an anxiety attack. I was feeling the impact of inner rage—fear out of control. I felt out of control. I panic every time I hear a jet fly overhead; I believe it is going to fall out of the sky and kill me. I am angry at God for letting it happen. The victims were innocent and vulnerable. I was innocent and vulnerable. They did not deserve to die like that. No one deserves to die like that. I am so sad and in so much pain. It is four months later and it still hurts so much."

I knew that anger was a normal emotion, but somehow this was an anger I could not control and it scared me. Some days the pain was so intense all I could feel was anger. Other days I felt nothing. I was emotionally numb. I felt robbed of a sense of purpose and passion. I was losing confidence in myself and my self-esteem was almost nonexistent.

As I struggled through each day, I tried to maintain my trust in the Lord. As days became weeks and weeks became months, the slow process of healing led to a deep depression. The depression was an awful place of profound sadness. Day after day there seemed to be no reason to get up or to go on. I cried a lot and was exhausted most of the time.

My life and my future were uncertain. I no longer felt safe in my world. Trauma survivors need to feel safe. Because of these feelings I could not continue to work, so five months after the event, I took a leave of absence. I was always fearful that I would have to respond to another disaster, and in my line of work this was not only possible, but probable. I hoped desperately that I could soon return to the work I loved. I found myself trying to do the things I used to do so routinely. I kept trying to be the person I was. This proved to be an effort in futility. That person was gone forever. I just didn't get it. I thought healing meant to return to who I was before the event. Realizing that a new path was a gift that I needed to receive was a concept that would take time to comprehend. It was far too early in the journey to take root.

I was on an emotional roller coaster and easily overwhelmed. One day, in January of '97, I went to the supermarket and as I approached the entrance, I froze. I stopped and held on to the shopping cart as if it were the only thing holding me together. I began to feel weak and dizzy and unable to move. I became disoriented and could not think of anything except that I had to get out of there immediately. Somehow I got to my car and made it home. I cried for a long time. I cried for the loss of so many innocent people; I cried for the loss of my innocence. Before the plane crash I was a high-functioning individual who could easily juggle five major projects at the same time. Now I could not even go food shopping without falling apart.

The intensity of my symptoms was not decreasing in fact it was getting worse. As a professional, I knew that the symptoms should begin to decrease within four to six weeks after the event. This is a key factor in determining if therapeutic intervention is needed. These signs and symptoms are all normal reactions initially; however, when they persist, PTSD may be a real consideration.

Feeling empty with nothing left inside, I literally dragged myself through the days and was plagued by sleepless nights. When I did sleep, the nightmares were haunting. I knew I needed professional help, but I found

myself resisting it. I couldn't believe my own bias. Fear
gripped my soul. What would people think? Pride reared
its ugly head. Would I be viewed as weak or even worse,
crazy? It was more than the loss of my career because I
was no longer able to work. It was my own perception of
who I was—who was I now and what did that mean? I
felt lost.

I would be the first person to recommend someone for
a referral if I felt they needed it. Now that it was me it was
a very scary place to be. I had to face the hard truth if I
were going to survive. This realization was a crucial
moment in my recovery. Was I willing to do whatever it
would take to get well? I was willing to try and for now
this would have to be good enough. Being willing and
trusting in the Lord would help me do the necessary leg
work to get the help I had to have. I sat quietly in the presence of Jesus. Just being with him. No words or petitions.
Just pure presence. Somehow the apostle Paul's words
became mine. "I can do all things through Christ who
strengthens me."

I recall the wisdom of Elizabeth-Ann Stewart who
wrote: "When catastrophe strikes, those who survive are
often left in a state of shock. Flood waters may subside,
raging fires may flicker out, bomb craters may be filled in,
but devastation continues its work in the minds and
hearts of those who have witnessed the unthinkable. No
one is exempted from traumatic stress; even counselors
and spiritual leaders wrestle with anger, fear and depression. Unnerved by their own experiences, they often find
it challenging to respond to others' anguish or to carry on
with their daily responsibilities; they, the 'healers' are

themselves in need of healing. In times of crisis, recovery is possible only when we return to our spiritual center. Though others may offer words of comfort and practical advice, it is God who keeps terror at bay, reassuring us that love is stronger than death, reminding us that we are not alone, no matter how dark the valley or how deep the abyss. When our world is shaken, God's house is the only place of refuge."

Understanding and support from loved ones, friends and colleagues can help tremendously during this time, and therapeutic intervention is often necessary.

Here are some suggestions for family and friends:

- Pray together. If your loved one is unable to pray— pray for them.
- Be prepared to be patient. Healing from trauma is a process not an event. It takes time to heal and each person has their own timetable.
- Spend time with the traumatized person.
- Reassure them they are safe.
- Offer your assistance and listen carefully to their needs.
- Send cards, flowers and call often.
- Help them with everyday tasks.
- Give them some space and private time.
- Don't tell them that they are "lucky it wasn't worse"— traumatized people are not consoled by those statements. Tell them that you are sorry such an event happened and that you want to understand and assist them.

- Don't take their anger or other feelings personally.
- Be in touch with your own needs and take care of yourself.

My anger was becoming a block to my relationship with Jesus Christ, my deepest spiritual resource. <u>How could I turn to a God I was so angry with.</u> I felt separated from God and I turned to scripture for answers and solace. "For he has not despised or disdained the suffering of the afflicted one; he has not hidden his face from him but has listened to his cry for help" (Psalms 22:24). I prayed that this was true.

∾ FOR REFLECTION ∾
"My Shaken World"

My world has been shaken Lord
There is no peace now,
In the waves that crest with bloody foam
Take me home

I don't want to feel this pain
So high the cost
This unfamiliar path is hard
Are you sleeping through my holocaust
Show me your face
Oh merciful God
For I am lost

You speak to my heart
Go within
It is there I dwell
It is there you begin

My journey will be long
For this I cry
Yet, you have given me living waters
Where I will never die
Because you are with me

Praise to You Lord, Jesus Christ

∞ AN INVITATION TO HEAL ∞

A RE the signs and symptoms of trauma affecting the quality of your life? Can you identify with any of those you have read about in this chapter? Are they persisting in time and severity? If so, then help is available. Only you can make the decision to seek help. It is a courageous step but a necessary one if you want to begin to feel better. We have mentioned a few initial steps you may want to consider.

- Prayer.
- Putting into place a support system.
- Sharing your story with a person you feel safe with.
- Identifying your signs and symptoms (see chart on pp. 54-55).
- Facing and feeling the pain in tolerable doses.
- Avoiding negative coping mechanisms such as alcohol and drugs.
- Engaging a trained mental health professional who has experience in treating trauma survivors.

COMMON SIGNS AND SYMPTOMS OF TRAUMATIC STRESS

PHYSICAL	COGNITIVE	EMOTIONAL	BEHAVIORAL	SPIRITUAL
Fatigue	Blaming someone	Anxiety	Less/more activity	Anger at God
Nausea	Confusion	Guilt	Change in speech patterns	Feeling distance from God
Muscle tremors	Poor attention	Grief	Withdrawal	Non-attendance at one's place of worship
Twitches	Poor decisions	Denial	Emotional outbursts	Uncharacteristic religious involvement
Chest pain*	Raised/lowered alertness	Emotional Shock	Suspiciousness	Sudden turn toward God
Difficulty breathing*	Poor concentration	Fear	Change in usual communication	Familiar faith practices seem empty (prayer, scriptures, hymns)
Elevated BP*	Memory problems	Uncertainty	Restlessness	Religious rituals seem empty (worship, communion)
Thirst	Hypervigilance	Severe Panic (rare)	Alcohol use increase	Doubting God's power
Headaches	Difficulty ID-ing familiar objects	Depression	Loss/increase in appetite	Loss of meaning and purpose

*indicates need for medical evaluation

COMMON SIGNS AND SYMPTOMS OF TRAUMATIC STRESS (Continued)

PHYSICAL	COGNITIVE	EMOTIONAL	BEHAVIORAL	SPIRITUAL
Visual problems	Flashbacks—intrusive images	Inappropriate Emotions	Acting out (antisocial behavior)	Sense of isolation (from God, religion, community)
Vomiting	Less awareness of surroundings	Apprehension	Nonspecific body complaints	Questioning of one's basic beliefs
Grinding Teeth (Bruxism)	Poor problem-solving ability	Feeling overwhelmed	Hyperalert to environment	Anger at clergy
Weakness	Reduced ability to think abstractly	Intense anger	Intensified startle reflex	Believing God is not in control
Dizziness	Loss of orientation	Irritability	Pacing	Believing God doesn't care
Profuse sweating	Impaired thinking	Agitation	Erratic movements	Belief that we have failed God
Chills and/or sweating, etc.	Nightmares		Increase/decrease in sexual drive	
Shock symptoms*				

*indicates need for medical evaluation

Questions for Reflection

1. Are you willing to participate in your recovery?

2. What will be your first step towards healing?

3. I invite you to begin by spending some time in silence with Jesus. While you are with him, what will you ask for?

5

Predisposition to PTSD

"Examination of the world without is never as personally painful as examination of the world within. Yet when one is dedicated to the truth, this pain seems relatively unimportant." —M. Scott Peck

PTSD is often understood to begin with a single excruciatingly stressful incident. Certainly that can be the case. However, it can also be caused by a series of traumatic or stressful encounters over a period of time. It never comes "out of the blue" but is the result of an overwhelming critical incident—either job related or personal. In addition, a person can sometimes be predisposed to the disorder from events that occurred much earlier in his or her life.

A predisposition to PTSD is based on several factors including:

1. Family History and Heredity
   From what I can remember and piece together from my mother's reminiscences, my father came home from World War II in 1945 with Post-Traumatic Stress Disorder. Of course, very little was known about

PTSD then so my father used the only source of pain relief that was socially acceptable: alcohol. He began drinking to wash away the horrors of war—to numb his pain. His symptoms revealed themselves in dangerous ways. Carrying me wrapped in a blanket, at only a couple of weeks old, he climbed a rope ladder on the side of a German ship docked in New York harbor. Despite the frantic pleading of my mother, he would not come down. He was reliving the war and it was just as real to him in that moment as it was when he was there. This irrational behavior almost cost both of us our lives.

My father's "startle reflex" (another sign of PTSD) was so raw that when my mother woke him in the morning for work he would fly out of the bed as if he had to escape a foxhole. Although he was frequently irritable, he managed to go to work sober every day. However, he would spend almost every weekend at the local bars—sometimes not coming home at all. When he was drinking he would relive the war. His closest friend had been blown up right next to him in the European theater. He was angry and when he was drinking he shouted out obscenities at the enemy. I remember as a child watching him sit in the living room openly sobbing. The alcohol anesthetized his pain and made it possible for him to express his anguish. His wound was bared so openly that it was frightening to be around him. Occasionally he would go into a rage and throw a chair across the room. He never hit me but I always lived in terror that he would. My wounds from living with an alcoholic were invisible and deep. A broken spirit can be just as painful as a broken arm.

I realize today how much pain my father lived with. I think of all soldiers who are living with PTSD and their families who are not getting the treatment they need. I pray for all of them. I pray the government will take care of all the men and women who put their lives on the line for all of us. And, if the government does not do their job, I challenge those who are hurting and those who love them to take charge and reach out for help. There is always hope.

2. Personal Trauma History

ACOA (Adult Children of Alcoholism) Growing up in an alcoholic environment I developed mistaken ideas about what was normal. What I thought was normal was not normal at all. This left me with numerous unresolved matters to deal with as an adult. Among these issues were broken trust, abandonment, lack of healthy communication skills, relationship problems and a struggle for intimacy. There was a child living inside of me who was never able to be a child. As an adult I needed to take her back so I could reclaim that part of my life.

Living with an alcoholic distorts one's ability to reason. It is difficult to develop a good sense of self since there was little praise for us as children. This fostered a desire in me to overachieve. It also caused me, as it often does in children who live in alcoholic homes, to form an overdeveloped sense of responsibility. I thought that having to do everything for everybody was normal. Somehow my siblings and I survived. My mother was a very spiritual woman and she had an unwavering faith in God. Her beautiful example of faith was highly instrumental in helping me form my own faith journey. I witnessed the peace she had through so much adversity, and I knew that it came from divine intervention—her peace did not come from this world.

"Then the peace of God, which is beyond all understanding, will guard your hearts and your minds in Christ Jesus" (Philippians 4:7). I wanted to know more about the peace she had so I began to pray more and I asked God to help me understand this peace. When I was in my early 40s I returned to church which I had been away from for many years. Coming back to the sheltering arms of God, I realized that He was never far from me all those years. It was I who turned from Him. I came to know that He is always faithful and by the power of his Holy Spirit I can heal and be transformed.

Through prayer and the merciful grace of Jesus I came to forgive my parents. The disease of alcoholism and its effects have been passed down to them, then to me and to my children in the form of the ACOA syndrome. My parents did the best they could have done at the time with the tools they had to work with. It is an intergenerational disease, but it can be treated. As the child of an alcoholic, I find great solace in that fact. I learned that I could no longer blame my parents for my life. I had to take responsibility for my own choices. With the help of an experienced alcoholism counselor and the Al-Anon and ACOA 12-step program, I was able to reclaim my childhood and move forward.

Divorce—I suffered the pain and trauma of divorce more than once. I knew I was not a bad person, so why couldn't I have a healthy marriage? During my time in counseling, I realized I had married my father twice. I had been recreating the dysfunction of my childhood family. I had no tools to perpetuate a healthy marriage—I didn't even know what one looked like. Divorce can be one of the most painful experiences a person will ever go through. It was for me. Yet through God's grace and healing love, while in counseling, I learned how to see myself as a whole and good person. Fear was replaced with peace.

Rape—This horrible trauma happened to me when I was in my twenties. Fearing for my life, I remember keeping the secret and the shame and guilt to myself. I was afraid of reporting it so I shut down my feelings and went on with my life. I know today that there is no such thing as just going on with your life after a personal trauma—left untreated it continues to affect your whole life. Some years later while working for the county and serving on a victim's rape committee, I did face my trauma. It was then I understood that rape is a crime of violence and it is never the victim's fault.

Motor Vehicle Accidents—As a teenager I left a party with my friend and her boyfriend, who had just bought a new car and was determined to show it off. Traveling at a high rate of speed, he missed a curve along the docks and plowed into a canal sinking five boats and his car. We were all pulled to safety by some neighbors who lived across the street from the canal. I was unconscious for a few minutes and I spent a few days in the hospital. Although I had no knowledge of it at the time, this was a very traumatic experience both physically and emotionally.

Recently a major research study, The Albany MVA Project, has identified some rather important findings in this area. Of the survivors of serious MVA's in which someone was injured sufficiently to require medical attention, 15% to 45% developed Post-Traumatic Stress Disorder immediately or within a year from the accident. Of the MVA survivors who developed PTSD:

— 53% to 78% develop severe depression

— 27% to 49% develop generalized anxiety disorder.

— 91% to 93% develop driving phobia.

(*After the Crash—Psychological Assessment & Treatment of Survivors of MVA*. Blanchard & Hickling, 2003.)

Sudden Death Loss—One of the most tragic events of my life was the loss of my three nephews who died in a fire in 1973. They were only two, three and four years old. They had stayed with me on Long Island for two weeks over the summer and they were home in Bay Port only three days when I received the heart-breaking news. It was so unreal. I kept thinking they were just here—how could they be gone? I sat on the couch and tried to gain some composure but I knew this wasn't going to happen any time soon. I was dazed and in shock and I didn't know what to do. The following day brought no relief. I kept remembering their little faces, their dazzling smiles and their laughter. And I remember the expressions on the faces of the firemen in the newspaper who carried their bodies, and the three little white coffins at the funeral.

Adding to my pain over the years, I had three close friends who died suddenly. One died at the early age of thirty in a car accident. Another was my partner while working in emergency services who was as close as a brother. At only thirty-one he died choking on food. A third close friend was a police officer who died in a diving accident while on vacation.

My own father also died suddenly of a heart attack. His death was really difficult for me because I had so much unfinished business with him. Fortunately, I was able to work through it and eventually I was able to say my good-byes. It is comforting to know that one can settle differences with loved ones who have died. My father died in 1976 and what I did not know at the time was that the pain I was going through was intensified by the symptoms of trauma. It would have been helpful to me if someone had been able to explain the trauma piece of my pain. Sometimes when we lose a loved one, we hold onto the pain because it's all we have left to connect us to them. The good news is that there is an end to the pain if we are willing to let go.

3. Career History
   A 27-year career in emergency medical services is the best description I have to define cumulative stress.

Facing trauma on a daily basis meant I was being exposed to many stressors over a long period of time—both job related and personal. Stress buildup happens slowly and often goes unrecognized and untreated. For this reason, every organization/Emergency service (paid or volunteer, military or civilian, private corporations, etc.,) needs to have a stress management education program in place for their employees. Stress awareness is an important factor in the physical and mental health of all people.

4. Events in your life one year prior to your trauma.
   These are the events that occurred in my life one year prior to the Flight 800 tragedy.
   Life Stress
   - my mother's death
   - an approaching marriage
   - birth of two grandchildren (both under very difficult emotional circumstances)
   - significant birthday (50)
   - the onset of menopause

   Job Stress
   - decision to retire from active field service (volunteer services).
   - Critical Incident Stress Management Team events—The team received some of the worst calls of its history that year. There were line of duty deaths, deaths of two chiefs' children, and two calls for murdered children. Those were just a few of the many calls, and I responded to over 50% of all calls.

- EMS—Many inter-office changes were taking place at my job with the county and there was a new medical director with a new administration.

I responded to and was in a leadership role in two major incidents:
- the wildfires of August 1995
- the blizzard of January 1996

These were some of the predisposing factors and stresses in my job and personal life just prior to the plane crash. Nothing could have prepared me for the disaster of that flight. Nothing could have prevented my heart from breaking or the chemistry in my body from changing as I witnessed unspeakable horror. We all have a threshold and sometimes the event is just too big to handle. I had to face this and accept that it changed my life. As Soren Kierkegaard described it so eloquently, "Life can only be understood backwards, but it must be lived forward."

Looking back, I could see the damaging effects of using negative coping mechanisms. Having lived with my father's alcoholism was a saving grace for me because it helped me make the choice not to go down that road. There is only one way through the pain and that is to face it, feel it and walk through it. It is the only way to get to the other side of it. With this knowledge I chose to bare my wounds in a safe and healthy way. It was now time for me to seek the professional help I needed.

∞ FOR REFLECTION ∞
"My History–My Teacher"

What have I learned
Through all the years
Joy and laughter
Suffering and tears
Much more than this
I am vulnerable but have not died
I am resilient and I can heal
I have limits
Yet with God, I can reach the stars
Through many dangers, toils and snares
I have already come
Amazing Grace indeed
Am I victim or survivor?
Simply
The one I feed.

∞ AN INVITATION TO HEAL ∞

What have you learned from the trauma you have survived?

Let's explore together the reality that God is the ultimate healing power, that prayer changes things and that God is faithful when we trust in His providence. We know Jesus was transformed by His passion of pain and suffering. With His grace we can be transformed also because it is never God's will for us to be in pain.

Consider the following:

• Awareness of the stress buildup in our lives can be the difference between health and sickness if we are willing to implement changes.

• Negative coping mechanisms are destructive.

• Taking responsibility for our lives and recovery is a choice.

• Blaming others for our circumstances keeps us stuck in denial.

• Keeping secrets about physical, sexual or emotional abuse can have a negative effect on a person's whole life. Abuse is never the victim's fault.

• Therapy and 12-step programs do work.

• Forgiveness is healing for the one who forgives. It begins with desiring to forgive and making a conscious decision to do so. Full forgiveness with the heart will come in time. It is often a process.

• The stages of grief are painful but necessary. Coupled with the symptoms of trauma, the process may be too overwhelming to handle alone. Professional help may be required.

• We can heal from the devastating events we encounter. Stay positive. Our present state of being is intimately connected and interwoven with our past experiences. Sometimes in the ruins of our past we can find direction for the future. Somewhere between these two places is the now, the present moment, where the Holy Spirit moves within and connects us to God, our spiritual center.

Questions for Reflection

1. How did you survive your past trauma?
2. How did God sustain you through it?
3. How can what you learned help you today?
4. Where is God present in your life today?

6

Seeking Help

"Therefore, I say to you, ask, and and it will be given you; seek, and you will find; knock and the door will be opened to you."   Luke 11:9

PTSD is the invisible wound. Shot by the invisible bullet I bled invisible blood. Even those closest to me did not know the depth of my pain. How could they? There were no obvious bruises, no bandages, no broken bones. How could anyone know? Yet I desperately needed someone to understand what I was going through.

Thomas the disciple of Jesus said, "Unless I see the mark of the nails in his hands and put my finger into the place where the nails pierced and insert my hand into his side, I will not believe" (John 20:25). Jesus was patient with Thomas. He let him touch his wounds. I also had to be patient with those around me. I had to let them touch my wounds if I wanted their understanding. I needed to let someone into my suffering. This very broken part of me that I was trying to hide had to be shared with someone with whom I felt safe.

I contacted a friend and colleague who worked with me on the CISM team as a leader for many years. Terry is a psychotherapist and teacher in the field of mental health and addictions. I knew, included in his training and experience, was treating PTSD. When we spoke on the telephone I told him what I was going through and that I was in a lot of pain. He urged me to come immediately so we could explore my treatment options. He was living in the Catskill mountains where he had established a healing and retreat center.

Driving three hours in my condition was a concern, but I knew God would be with me every mile. I set out for the mountains the following morning and the trip, as I trusted, was uneventful. When I reached the house, the door was open and I could smell the lovely fragrance of burning incense. In the background a Gregorian Chant was playing and the peace that I had lost began to return. As Terry emerged from the kitchen of the twenty-two bedroom house and reached out to embrace my pain-riddled body, the long awaited tears began flowing. Over a cup of tea I talked about the plane crash and tears rolled down my face like a gentle waterfall. I was feeling a deep sense of relief in response to his understanding and empathy. My inner fear and discomfort had lessened a great deal and I felt more hopeful.

The next day we started our work. My feelings were very raw, so we decided I would participate in the Art of Loving Experiential Retreat that was starting that weekend. I had attended one before so I had a point of reference for it. Feelings have a central place in this model with special attention focused on suppressed fears, anger, grief and pain as they block the flow of free-flowing energy. Over the next few days we used Gestalt, Bioenergetics, primal scream, physical expulsion of anger and role play. One of the strengths of this model is that it allows the person to evolve at his/her own pace. It works with whatever a person's issues are in that moment (fear, loss, anger, etc.) and keeps the individual in the present by making a variety of tools, resources and options available in a very safe, supportive and encouraging environment. I was able to release a lot of emotional energy as well as allow adequate time for processing, soothing and comforting. These were all things I was not able to do in an emergency situation. On the last day of the retreat I was feeling even more hopeful for my future. I left for home with renewed energy and a deep sense of gratitude for Terry and his love

Because I had worked with trauma survivors for many years, I knew the importance of finding a therapist who had both training and experience in treating psychological trauma. I would not go to a podiatrist for a cardiac problem, and I also would not settle for just any therapist. Trauma injury presents very specific needs so I was determined to find appropriate treatment. I was feeling the crippling effects of low self-esteem and depression so I moved slowly at first. Decision-making was arduous, yet I was able to move forward and interview two therapists. One lacked experience in treating PTSD, and I was not comfortable with the personality of the other. I respected my own personal needs and kept seeking.

Eventually I remembered a psychologist I met several years before at a trauma conference. I contacted him and after we spoke I felt sure he was a clinician I could work with. I trusted him. Trust is a very important ingredient in the doctor/patient relationship. Besides his extensive training and experience in treating PTSD, he also possessed the spiritual component I was looking for—he was comfortable with my talking about my faith. Our rapport was crucial for my recovery. I saw no signs of bias or sexism. These negating characteristics can leave a patient feeling guilty or full of shame. I felt I had made a good decision which helped me to feel like I had some control over my life again. In turn it helped to increase my self-esteem. Also by taking this step I was acknowledging that my injury was real. That acceptance came slowly as my own prejudice was exposed and overcome—none of which I wanted to face. I wanted to be ok. To fit in. To feel whole once again.

We began meeting twice a week, and I was now feeling secure enough to take another step in my recovery. I discussed with Dr. B. my feelings about attending the On-Site-Academy in Gardner, Massachusetts which is a not-for-profit organization dedicated to the health and well-being of all emergency services personnel and their families. It is an in-house five-day critical incident stress program geared to emergency services personnel who are themselves temporarily overwhelmed by the stress of their jobs—what they have seen, and what they have been through. The care includes training in managing post-trauma symptoms, individual and group therapy, EMD-R (Eye Movement Desensitization Reprocessing), and peer support counseling. With his support and encouragement I went to the Center and participated in this training plan. The time I spent there turned out to be instrumental in my recovery because it helped me to rebuild my foundation of stability that had crumbled beneath me under the extreme and prolonged stress of Flight 800. The treatment I received there from Dr. Hayden Dugan, Valerie Dugan and all of the peer counselors was professional, sensitive and effective. I will always be grateful to them for their dedication to helping others heal.

After my stay at the On-Site-Academy, I returned to Long Island and resumed therapy. I was on leave from my job now for about a month and was not ready to go back. I was determined to recover, and yet the reality was maybe I could never go back. My main goal was to get back to the work I so dearly loved. It was my life. It was who I was.

Therapy was going along well, yet my anxiety and depression were still very difficult to live with. The possibility of taking medication made me feel like I had somehow failed in my progress. I took some time with this decision because that feeling of "if I have to take medication then I must not be ok" was playing again. Also I was afraid of the side effects of the medication. I did not realize at the time what a great help medication can be and how it can actually enhance the positive effects of therapy. Dr. S., a psychiatrist with excellent credentials, suggested I take an anti-anxiety/antidepressant medication. He fully explained how the medication worked, and the possible side effects. He answered every question I asked without hesitation and I liked the idea that we would move slowly. Assuring me that it was my decision to take the medication, he left the door open for me to call him whenever I needed to. He was caring, patient, honest and informative—all the qualities I needed to help me move through my fear.

I chose to take the medication and at first I felt a little disconnected, but that soon passed and I began to feel better. I thanked God for helping me to take this step. I came to understand that therapy and medication are tools God gives us to heal. There are many people with confirmed diagnosis for which therapy and medication could be of great assistance. In some cases it can mean the difference between living in chaos and pain or living healthy, productive lives. I know the feeling of shame that stigmas impose but after awhile I no longer accepted the world and its stigmas as my own. I wanted to get better for myself and my family.

Soon I realized that the Lord has always seen me as ok—as whole. I came to this understanding when I started to see a spiritual director. Working with Annette proved to be a very special time for me. She is truly a channel for the Holy Spirit. Her ministry is a testimony of miracles. Through prayer and her presence I was able to talk about the plane crash on a very deep feeling level. Sometimes I would sob uncontrollably. She listened and let the tears flow. My pain touched her but did not interfere with her guidance. The peace I received was divine in nature. Soon I realized that I could not find God in my pain, but I found Him in my surrender. Once again the Lord sent me what I needed. Once again He gave me the courage to do what I needed to do to heal. Spiritual direction together with therapy and medication provided healing for my body, mind and spirit.

We need to be willing to seek and knock, and the door will be opened unto us.

∞ FOR REFLECTION ∞

"The Gifted Healers"

They walked the road with one so broken,
In quiet wisdom their words were spoken.
Time dear friend would be a wonder,
A statement made and left to ponder.

Many feelings would have to be faced,
Grief, abandonment and even disgrace.
None would cause the pain so deep,
As the lost ministry I could not keep.

Winter, summer, spring and fall,
Gifted healers saw me through them all.
Endless waiting, endless pain,
Ever hopeful they remained.

I always knew that I was heard,
Especially when joined by the divine third.
The Holy Spirit guided every session,
Lifting in His time the deep depression.

Time has passed, work has been done.
A new life is emerging, a new life has begun.
Caregivers to my wounded soul,
Because of you today I am whole.

∞ AN INVITATION TO HEAL ∞

SOME things to consider when seeking therapy:

• You are the consumer. Explore all resources (therapists, treatment centers, support groups, spiritual direction, etc.)

• Educate yourself about your injury.

• Interview therapists and ask questions about their credentials, education and training as well as their experience in treating trauma survivors.

• Tune into your own needs. Listen to your intuition and trust your needs will be met.

• Assess any existing secondary problems such as addictions, depression, etc. The more you know about yourself the more you will be able to help your therapist to help you.

• Let others share your pain. Let them touch your wounds.

• Don't quit no matter how bad it seems. Stay with it. You will get better. God is faithful.

The healing process may be a long journey but it does not have to be lonely. In prayer we petition the Lord and his compassionate healers to walk this path with us.

Questions for Reflection

1. Can you let others share your pain?
2. Are you in touch with your own needs?
3. What are they, and how will you fulfill them?

7

In the Present Moment

" When I awaken, I will be blessed by beholding you."
Psalms 17:15

ONE day life is going along smoothly and in the blink of an eye we experience a traumatic event. Feeling lost and confused, we find we are left with a shattered belief system. We know life has changed and that we are not feeling ok, but it may never occur to us that we cannot get through this nightmare alone. In time it becomes clear that we need to reach out for help. Time alone does not heal PTSD. It takes time plus therapy and a relationship with and trust in the Holy Spirit. I found these three factors were critical to my healing process.

1. Time—Trauma is ultimately connected to loss, but does not only refer to losing a loved one. During my recovery I had to endure the grief process over and over again. Allowing time was important because each of my losses revealed themselves at different times. I lost my health, my sense of safety and well-being, my life's work and financial security. Most importantly, I lost my identity (who I was before the trauma), and my social structure

which was my EMS family. I could never have dealt with all this at once. The symptoms, triggers and losses combined were too overwhelming to process them all at the same time. It had to be sorted out slowly and with help.

Time is also essential because it allows for continuity. After my trauma I lost my sense of orientation. I lost my bearings on what made sense to me, and I needed my therapist to help me take a step back and look at the present moment. I found myself worrying about the future and that was non-productive and self defeating. As quoted by Dr. Bessel Van der Kolk, at the Psychological Trauma Conference, Boston, MA in 2007, "PTSD is an illness of not being able to stay in the present." Dwelling on past trauma and worrying about the future was blocking my recovery. However, in therapy I was able to keep life in perspective one day at a time. Staying in the present was not always easy but eventually it gave me the power to take control of my life again.

2. Opening Up to the Help of Others—Once I was able to trust my therapist and the therapeutic process, I found my daily life was beginning to be more stable. I had lost a lot of my coping mechanisms, and now, with help, I was building new ones as I dealt with the triggers of past and present trauma. I was grateful to have someone to help me stay in the present and sort out the triggers and the reactions. Together we were building strategies for self-esteem and renewed confidence both from within and from outside influences. Safety is crucial for one who is dealing with PTSD, and I felt safe in this relationship. This trust builds over time and there is value in the process.

Each time I reached out I did so from a better place, a place of deeper healing. I moved forward slowly and even when I fell back I learned from my therapist that it was ok because it is a normal part of healing. So staying in the present became my lifeline.

3. Opening Up to the Holy Spirit—PTSD was an injury to my very soul. The suffering was beyond my understanding. This pain caused me to open up my heart to the Holy Spirit in a way that brought me closer to the Spirit. I am grateful to have had the chance to go so deeply within to find my true self. Once I was dead to my old self, I was able to create the space for the Spirit to enter. As quoted by John of the Cross "If we were perfectly dead to ourselves . . . then might we be able to relish things divine." Death to self leaves us open to trust in God's grace. This was the beginning of the healing of my spiritual life.

My therapist was careful to work within my comfort zone to protect me from being re-traumatized and triggering any PTSD symptoms. In time and with the power of the Holy Spirit we discovered each new path as we went along. The path or road map for recovery was already formed—I just needed to surrender myself to the Spirit. This eventually led me to experience emotional freedom and pointed me towards a life of greater meaning. I was learning that the present moment was not such a bad place to be and that I could survive and even live very nicely there. Practicing contemplative prayer was a great help to me at this time. It felt good to slow down my life and to learn how to just "be" with the Spirit. I found myself meditating on the things of God. I sought out gardens and beautiful places where nature's abundance brought me peace. Getting in touch with my spiritual self was a major factor in my quest for patience and patience is simply peace while waiting. Ultimately it is all connected by the Holy Spirit.

∞ FOR REFLECTION ∞

"A Prayer of Gratitude"

Thank you, Lord, for the gift of time.
May I always use it wisely to fulfill your purpose for my life.

Thank you, Lord, that I have come to accept that all things happen in your time, not mine.

Thank you, Lord, for the gift of therapy and my therapist.
I will always be grateful for his patience and skill.
I trust one day, Lord, you will greet him with these words, "Well done good and faithful servant."

Thank you, Lord, for the gift of the Holy Spirit.
May I always live in the fullness of that spirit and use these gifts to help others.

Thank you, Lord, for a heart full of gratitude.

∞ AN INVITATION TO HEAL ∞

LETTING go of one way of life and learning to live another way can be as exciting and interesting as it is painful and confusing. As a new direction and new interests begin to form we can begin to see little everyday miracles start to unfold. When your heart gets lighter and pain begins to fade, I invite you to put your trust in the Holy Spirit and let a new joy begin to take hold within your spirit.

When you awaken each day there will be two choices before you. You can either do your very best to make it a good day or you can stay stuck in pain. The choice is yours. Remember the Holy Spirit cannot do the work *for* you—only *with* you. This requires you to let go of your old beliefs so you may start to build new ones and come to know your own truths. You need to let go of shame and fear and take courage in the hope of a new day.

Today I walk with a psychological limp, yet I trust that God uses all things for the good. If you do not know the Holy Spirit, I invite you to introduce yourself and take notice of all the wonders the Spirit will grace you with.

Will you pray with me?

"Holy Spirit I welcome you into my life today. Help me to rest quietly with you and fill me with your precious love. I want to know it more, so I can bring it to everyone I meet. I am so grateful that you have embraced me with your faithfulness."

Questions for Reflection

1. Are you open to receiving the joy of the Holy Spirit?
2. Where is the Holy Spirit leading you?

8

A Safe Place

"For the greater glory of God"

—St. Ignatius Loyola

MY therapy was going well but I felt the need for something more. My therapist was extremely helpful and my family was loving, yet there was a deep longing for a supportive spiritual community. It seemed there was a hole in my chest, one that could only be filled by a relationship with Jesus Christ. Because of the interruption in the life I knew, I suffered the pain of feeling abandoned by friends and co-workers. I had to face the fact that I was disabled. As inconceivable as this concept was to me, I could not ignore the evidence that I had gathered for the disability hearings.

The confusion and inner turmoil were devastating. It was only by the power of the Holy Spirit that I made it to the hearings. My financial survival depended on my disability pension being approved. God answered my prayers and gave me the strength I needed to get through this difficult time.

The loss of my sense of community added to my distress. The truth is, friends I had worked with for years did stand by me, but the time came when they had to go on with their lives. This is a normal progression, and as painful as it was I had to let them go. Holding on to them and who I used to be as a rescuer caused me additional pain and became a block in my healing process. I was disabled and would have to come to terms with that before my recovery could continue.

A friend told me about a place in Plainview, NY called the Spirit Life Center. It was the ministry of a Jesuit priest, Reverend Robert McGuire—a tall, soft spoken, gentle man. I knew the first time I met Fr. Bob that he had a unique understanding and compassion for his flock. Many injured souls would find themselves on his doorstep—myself included. All were welcome, and one's affliction didn't matter. So many came, the physically handicapped, as well as the mentally, emotionally and spiritually broken. No one was judged or turned away.

Walking through the doors of the Spirit Life Center, a feeling of peace came over me which is hard to explain. It was surely Holy Ground. I trusted in my heart that it was a good place. This was a ministry dedicated to, and a manifestation of the Holy Spirit and the healing power of Jesus. It was an expression of the maternal love of the Church reaching out to her wounded people. Through Spirit Life I found comfort and healing, drawing on the strength of a Christian community which came together in praise, Eucharistic prayer, and instruction. There is no doubt that my being there was in direct response to God's invitation for me to heal. He led me to the community of Spirit Life Center and the wisdom of Father Bob. I rejoice with St. Paul: "Blessed be the God and Father of our Lord

Jesus Christ, the Father of mercy and the God of all consolation. He consoles us in all our afflictions and thereby enables us to console others in their tribulations . . ."(2 Corinthians 1:3-4).

There were times when my self-esteem was so low all I could do was isolate. Isolation can appear in the form of a blessing initially. There is no one there to put demands on you, no one to judge you or to put their expectations on your life and progress. It feels good to be left alone, even peaceful. There are times when we need that for a little while; however too much isolation can become a negative coping mechanism. By staying alone too much, I would lose my sense of a healthy perspective on life. My thinking became negative and fear would rule the days. Depression would take hold and it was a downward spiral until I forced myself to reach out to people. I learned the phone worked two ways and I had to use it, too. Just as quickly as I went into the darkness, I found it could be reversed by reaching out to a friend, therapist, spiritual director, or going to my Al-Anon meeting or spiritual community for support. Hope in the darkness is a choice and in the midst of it all, there is God.

Father Bob had a goal. He believed I could heal. He would ask me to do small tasks. First it was sharpening pencils. Then hanging pictures, and on to cleaning the kitchen after lunch. He asked me to do some cooking and was advised this was not one of my gifts. After one meal he saw the light. We moved on to setting the altar before Mass. The memory of feeling great humility and a sense of grace while performing this task is still with me. Who was I to touch the instruments of the holy Mass? My knowledge of how much God loved me was growing. With encouragement and the completion of each new task my self-esteem grew and I began to feel better about myself. This was a slow process. Soon, however, love and patience with myself became a natural response for me.

One day Father Bob suggested I become one of the facilitators for the mini retreat—a weekly scripture sharing event. As a facilitator I would have to sit in front of the group and start the day with prayer and introductions. After the scripture of the day is read, individuals share their own experience of how the Word is working in their lives. Fr. Bob's request to lead the group surprised me. I wanted to run away; fear gripped me. This was a strange reaction coming from someone who once conducted meetings effortlessly. I realized that it was hitting too close to home—doing the one thing by which I was so injured when I was doing the critical incident stress debriefings after the Flight 800 disaster. It is a good example of how PTSD can destroy our self-confidence. With Fr. Bob's continued encouragement, I gave it a try and did well. I found that it was very different from the debriefings. We were gathered on holy ground and in a peaceful atmosphere where people could share their pain and learn that God's Word was alive and active. I soon discovered that the gifts I used on my job while companioning others who had known trauma could still help people. Only now something was different. I had met Jesus, the Wounded Healer, on a new level. The depth of my pain was turning me into a wounded healer. Who can take away suffering without first entering in? Jesus, in his passion, entered into our pain. He has sent the Holy Spirit to continue this work in all of us of healing our wounds so that we can use that knowledge and experience to help others. To enter in.

Each time I said yes, I came closer to letting go of my past and my pain. The lesson I learned is never to put limitations on God. As Father Bob watched my transformation into a self-assured wounded healer he asked me to give a seminar at the Center for trauma survivors. I thought about it, and with much trepidation, said yes. This was the beginning of a fuller dimension of my previous work because this time Jesus' wounds and mine had touched.

At Spirit Life I experienced a new sense of belonging: a place where the Holy Spirit dwelled; a place that filled my heart. The mini retreat was a healing experience, and meditating, reflecting and sharing on the Word of God was profound because now I was drawing on His strength and healing love. The people who attended the mini retreat encouraged me and accepted me just the way I was. We grew into a community of God's power and love. If I had said no to these many opportunities for healing, moving on might never have happened.

One of the wonderful programs at the Spirit Life Center which was particularly helpful to me was the Adult Child of the King (ACOK) a 12-step support group that recognized Jesus Christ as our higher power. I no longer thought of myself as the child of an alcoholic. Through this program I learned I was the child of a king. What a concept! Do you know what it means to be the child of a king? Can you imagine being so special? In this loving community I was able to accept my brokenness because I felt safe and loved.

There will always be gratitude in my heart for that gentle spirited Jesuit who had a vision and followed it. His ministry at the Spirit Life Center helped me and so many others heal through the integration of spirituality, therapeutic process, the power and grace of the sacraments and the freedom and opportunity to experience the movement of the Holy Spirit. Today, by the power of God's love, I am more trusting that my life and ministry are a testimony to the greater glory of God.

∞ FOR REFLECTION ∞

"Movement of the Holy Spirit"

Fleeting is the moment
When the human spirit connects
With the divine

SUDDENLY

Just as leaves dance upon the wind
You enter my being
With the softness of a gentle summer breeze
My heart is stirred
Your love embraces my soul
Peace abides within

PRESENCE

Pure Holy Presence
We touch
I am loved
Fleeting is the moment
Eternal is the union
Sacred, Holy and from God

∞ AN INVITATION TO HEAL ∞

Light and Shadow
  are opposite sides of the same
  coin. We can illuminate our paths or
  darken our way.
    It is a matter of choice.

—Maya Angelou

TO illuminate our path may mean taking some risks. Like taking a leap of faith and moving out of our comfort zone. Becoming part of a spiritual community may feel like that leap of faith, but it may also be the beginning of hope in the darkness. Given the opportunity it is likely to become a very concrete part of your healing journey.

Listed below are some of the attributes of a prayerful community where God's children gather in an atmosphere of spiritual freedom.

• a time and place to pray and seek a deeper relationship with God

• safety to embrace our own brokenness

• encouragement to draw on God's love and strength and to openly receive it

• an opportunity to be with spiritual people and have a new sense of belonging

• courage to say yes to new experiences and not put limits on God

• confidence to be patient and gentle with ourselves and to learn to trust again

Most faith-based organizations of all denominations offer some form of spiritual support groups. I invite you to illuminate your path by seeking a community in which you can grow in wisdom and grace.

Questions for Reflection

1. Are you willing to take a risk and work for inner harmony?
2. How balanced is your life today?
3. Are you open to the movement of the Holy Spirit in your life?

9

Tools for Recovery

"Fear not, beloved, you are safe; take courage and be strong."   Daniel 10:19

IF we build the courage to pick up these tools, then we can count on the power of God to move us out of the darkness and into the light. In my reflection in chapter 3 God promised to call me out of the tomb. He also told me I would learn from Him there. In the darkness and the stillness a complete death to self and ego took place, followed by a profound nothingness. I waited to feel better, to heal and to move forward. During this time a transformation from within me took place. Just as I went to the cross with Jesus, I was now beginning to experience the promise of the resurrection. With God's grace and the tools He gave me, I have built a bridge between the crucifixion and the resurrection, between darkness and light, despair and hope.

When He called me out of the tomb, He was telling me that my suffering was not the end but a passage to new life. I needed only to pick up the tools and use them. It was a joint effort—God and me.

1. *Prayer*—Prayer is a wonderful way to build a relationship with God because prayer is conversation with God. There are many ways to pray. Sometimes we talk to God or ask for His help and sometimes we are called into solitude just to listen. Meditation and contemplation in His presence are very calming and peaceful. There is a merciful and all-forgiving God longing for you to come into His friendship. Lovingly He gazes upon your soul waiting to give you life. Prayer and your relationship with God become your first line of healing and a graced way of life.

2. *Willingness to Participate in the Recovery Process*—God has given us a free will. He doesn't interfere with that free will. It is our choice to seek healing or to stay a victim. It is because of my willingness to ask the Lord for His help and to use these tools that I am able to reach out to you today and offer you hope. Life for me has been transformed in my surrender, but I had to use the tools and work through the process.

3. *A Safe Place*—After experiencing a trauma, one of our most essential needs is to feel safe. Initially I felt safe with my therapist. Once we built that foundation of trust, I was able to slowly expand my comfort zone. The safety we need may come in different ways for each of us. It could be your home where there is support from family or a club or organization where you have support from friends and co-workers. Perhaps it is a place of worship or spiritual community. Maybe it is a twelve-step group. Wherever you feel safe and supported is your safe place.

4. *Education about PTSD*—When something affects us that we do not understand, it can be very frightening

and confusing causing a lot of anxiety. Often just knowing the facts about PTSD can offer a clear picture of what is happening to us. Also it can give us direction and show us how to get help. The library has many books on the subject; the internet also has a lot of information. Talking with an experienced therapist can help. This education needs to include family and all those closest to you.

5. *Therapy/Medication*—Therapy and sometimes medication are paramount for treating the injury of PTSD. PTSD cannot be handled alone. Help is there just waiting for you to reach out and ask for it. Remember trauma is a specialty. You can contact your local mental health services for direction. The final choice of a therapist is yours.

6. *Support Groups*—Support groups are a great adjunct to therapy. Joining a group helps decrease the sense of being alone. Isolation is non-productive in the treatment of PTSD. In a group others are struggling along with you. You can laugh and cry together and you understand why. You can check with your therapist for information concerning therapeutic support groups. Others may include faith-based community groups, bereavement groups, AA, Al-Anon or other 12-step groups. While I was on this long journey I used almost all of them.

7. *Expressing Our Feelings*—A very positive part of healing from trauma is to be aware of how we are feeling. Remember feelings are not right or wrong. They just are. It is what we do with them and how we express them that is important. For example, when strong feel-

ings such as anger arise, do we start an argument with a family member or go for a long run or to the gym? Our emotions can be dealt with in a healthy and loving way. Some ways that may help are: talking about how we are feeling, journaling, painting, writing poetry, physical activity, etc. These are just a few ways to lessen the intensity of our feelings by working through them.

8. *Feeling Our Feelings*—There is no magic wand that will quickly take away the pain of trauma symptoms, grief and loss. There are times when we will just need to let ourselves feel. Our human nature is to run from pain. But understand that pain is a great motivator and teacher. Your courage to endure this process will have great rewards. To the extent that you let yourself feel the pain, will be the extent you will feel joy and healing. Allow yourself to feel the feelings. They will not annihilate you.

9. *Waiting*—Sometimes we just have to let go and give our life over to God. One day at a time I could let go of who I was. In the waiting there is healing. In the waiting is becoming and learning wisdom. It is not easy, but it is necessary. In Psalm 13 the psalmist cries out, "How long, O Lord—will you forget me forever?" It can feel like the Lord has abandoned us. Trust that He has the whole picture and we do not. In His time He will show you His purpose for your life. Life has changed as it was, not ended.

10. *Pet Therapy*—our animal friends can be a wonderful source of comfort. My beautiful and gentle Akita was at times my therapist just by her unconditional love

and presence. She was my friend and faithful companion and an intricate part of my healing journey. She went home to the Lord on December 27, 2005, but she will always be in my heart.

11. *Accepting Limitations*—This is a grief process and it happens over time. There was an initial period of deep sadness for all the losses. Eventually I began to focus on gratitude. I realized that acceptance brought me peace by letting God do what I could not do. This did not happen easily and sometimes it was extremely difficult. In life we will always have to accept changes that we may not like. Accepting our limitations does not defeat us, but frees us.

12. *Exercise, Nutrition, Rest and Relaxation*—Do we reverence our body, the vehicle in which we live? I could write a book about each of the above topics, but I simply want to emphasize that health of mind goes hand in hand with a healthy body. The whole person concept includes our physical, mental, emotional, social and spiritual selves. They all need our attention and care, both collectively and individually. When the total person is functioning at full capacity and in balance, then we have taken one more step towards health and wholeness. We become the true creation of God, fully His, fully alive.

13. *Doing Things That Bring You Joy*—What makes you feel good—travel, hiking, reading, rock climbing, concerts, retreats, prayer, meditation or taking walks on the beach? Whatever it is, do it often. We need to offset the stress in our lives with pleasure and fun. Play and laughter are food for the soul. A good laugh can offset

the gut-wrenching pain we feel during recovery. At times it was only my sense of humor that kept me going.

14. *Taking Risks*—We take a risk in response to our pain or needs. Each time I picked up one of these tools I was responding to some need within me. At times just baby steps were taken but it was a start. With each step I asked the Lord to walk with me. Soon the baby steps became giant steps. Moving out of my comfort zone enabled me to heal and grow.

As I continued to use these tools, I found my life was beginning to fall into balance. I did my part and God, who is always faithful, did His. It became evident to me that on a daily basis I was beginning to identify and listen to my needs. This takes practice, especially for a rescuer who generally puts the needs of others first. If I was tired, I rested. If I needed to talk, I called my therapist or a friend. If I felt overwhelmed, I took my dog and walked along the beach. If I felt the need to be close to Jesus, I found a quiet place and put myself in his presence. Slowly I realized life can be good again. I needed this time to learn how to love and care for myself. This is something God has always wanted for me, but I was too wounded to hear Him over my own ego.

If we can use these tools on a regular basis and in a balanced way, then I truly believe that God will reveal His purpose for each of us. Believe and move forward to the reward that awaits you.

∞ FOR REFLECTION ∞

One ship drives east and another drives west
With the self same winds that blow.
'Tis the set of the sails
And not the gales,
That tells us the way to go.

Like the winds of the sea are the ways of fate;
As we voyage along through life.
'Tis the set of the soul
That decides its goal,
And not the calm or the strife.

—Ella Wheeler Wilcox

∞ AN INVITATION TO HEAL ∞

I INVITE you to walk with us—God and me. The path that I have walked has been revealed to you. In this book I have shared with you my pain, grief, loss and also my faith journey from victim to survivor to healer. When we are lost in the forest, God sends a guide. When we do not know the way, He sends a navigator. Very often our guide comes in the form of another person—someone who has already been where we are but has made it through the forest. It may be someone who has found a path or someone who has made it across the rope bridge onto solid ground. It may be someone like me or you who has picked up the tools for healing and used them. The insights found in using these tools can make the road we are walking seem straighter, the pain less heavy and eventually the light more real and attainable. It is always easier when we walk with someone who has traveled through the darkness. My friend, I have been there and my hope for you is that by my witness of using these tools, you too will find healing and peace.

It is offered to you as pure gift. With love from God and me.

Questions for Reflection

1. What tools are you using to assist you on your journey?

2. Who are your guides?

10

Transformation

"He himself bore our sins in His body upon the cross, so that, free from sin we might live for righteousness. By His wounds you have been healed."

1 Peter 2:24

⚬⚮⚬

LIFE is full of change on many levels, but true transformation can only happen by embracing the suffering and taking many risks. While on this healing journey I did not turn to those who would only offer comfort to my old self. I had to literally risk my whole self, to endure suffering and pass courageously through it, making it a faith-filled rite of passage through the wounds of Jesus Christ.

It is by the union of his sacred wounds with ours that we are transformed. When our wounds are healed, they become sacred wounds. After the resurrection, Jesus returned with his wounds. Can we accept that the risen Jesus is also the wounded Jesus? Are there wounds in your life that still need healing? Are you open to allow healing to take place? Are you willing to face what may feel like annihilation so that the soul which is indestructible within you can live and be transformed? These are questions of the soul and we need to go within for the answers.

Jesus rose from death and continues to teach us, heal us and to breathe his peace into our souls. He sends us forth in his name to feed his sheep—to be a binder of wounds and healer of hearts.

When we are transformed into whole and holy people, bound to Jesus in salvation and sanctification, we are a glorious extension of the true purpose for our lives—to serve God and each other. We companion one another across the threshold of the earthly life into eternal life, while leaving behind the fear, anxiety, isolation and pain. We shed all that is not of God right here on earth.

The mystery of the inner life causes us to seek higher levels of consciousness in our feeling, thinking and acting. This higher level of consciousness can be attained through our relationship with Jesus and our walk with him through his Passion, Death and Resurrection. ". . . and if children, then heirs, heirs of God and joint heirs with Christ. If only we suffer with Him so that we may be glorified with Him" (Rom 8:17). Only when we go beyond the fear of annihilation, as Jesus did on the cross, can our contact with the divine begin and the promise of new life in Christ be achieved. He is calling us to serve others in this life, but ultimately he is calling us to peace, healing, love, joy and happiness.

He is calling us home to himself and to eternal life.

∞ FOR REFLECTION ∞

Oh joy, you elusive delight
How you have evaded me in the dark hours
I see you there peeking through the fading shadow
Come closer I am ready to meet you

My heart is open, filled with hope
You have been there all the time
The clouds have lifted
I can see and feel you now

How glorious your gift
Truly life giving
I feel the dawn of a new day
Deep In my soul

How great is our God
Who is faithful to His promises
To your unconditional love
I respond with gratitude

I have been to the cross with you
Now I am living in the joy of resurrection
Thank you Jesus!

∞ AN INVITATION TO HEAL ∞

I INVITE you to use this scripture for reflection and sharing.

"Trust wholeheartedly in the Lord
rather than relying on your own intelligence.

In everything you do, acknowledge Him,
and He will see that your paths are straight."

Proverbs 3:5-6

Questions for Reflection

1. In what ways can you trust in the Lord and surrender your will to him?

2. Do you allow him to direct your path?

CONCLUSION

Living Resurrection

"For I know the plans I have for you declares the Lord, plans to prosper you and not to harm you, plans to give you hope and a future. —Jer 29:11

TODAY I walked along the peaceful shore and as I watched a beautiful butterfly come to rest on my shoulder, all the world fell silent. Without explanation I knew I was in the presence of God. There was a holy stillness within my soul. Perhaps beyond my soul? I found I had a thirst that could only be quenched by being with the God of my creation in a place of eternal fellowship. I felt in these moments I was experiencing the resurrection of Jesus and was being given a taste of our promised eternal happiness. Perhaps a tiny peek into the eternal? With no further explanation than this astounding moment in time, I began to reflect on what God's purpose for my life is today. How was I already living the joys of the resurrection right here on earth?

Since my injury and in the process of my healing there has been a lot of growth in my person, my faith and in my spirit. Hence, God uses all things for the good. The Lord has given me many gifts and in this time he has been pruning me and strengthening me to be sent forth in His name to help those who are still suffering and who are lost in the darkness. He has no hands here now but ours so it is with great joy that I am able to serve God's people. As I ponder this reality, I see how the Lord has orchestrated my future according to His purpose.

Today I am a trained spiritual director and I companion people who are recovering from trauma. I do this in spiritual direction and through workshops, seminars and retreats on healing from trauma and PTSD. I have shared my story in this book and have given talks in retreat centers, churches, colleges, etc. I can talk about my wounds without fear and answer any question with a spirit of courage and honesty.

I am grateful to God my Father that I am becoming the person He made me to be. I trust He will continue to renew me in His spirit so my life may always reveal the reality of Jesus' resurrection.

Relying on God's infinite love to heal all those who turn to Him in need, I encourage you to have faith and trust in the Lord. My friends, I know He will never abandon you in your time of need.

RESOURCES

- If you are suffering from the wounds of post-traumatic stress,

- If you are a parent, spouse, family member or friend who wants more information to understand and help someone suffering from PTSD,

- If you are in any way concerned with the healing of PTSD,

this Resource Guide will help you. Please refer to it for a variety of useful materials.

Author

The author invites you to write her at:

> P.O. Box 828
> Medford, NY 11763

Books

Antoinette Bosco. *Shaken Faith: Hanging in There When God Seems Far Away.* New London, CT: Twenty-third Publications, 2001.

Monique Lang. *Healing from Post-Traumatic Stress.* New York: McGraw Hill, 2007.

Peter A. Levine. *Waking the Tiger: Healing Trauma.* Berkeley, CA: North Atlantic Books, 1997.

Dalene C. Fuller Rogers. *Pastoral Care for Post-Traumatic Stress Disorder: Healing the Shattered Soul.* New York: Haworth Press, 2002.

Dena Rosenbloom, Mary Beth Williams. *Life After Trauma: A Workbook for Healing.* NewYork: The Guilford Press, 2000.

Glenn R. Schiraldi. *Post-Traumatic Stress Disorder Sourcebook.* Lincolnwood, IL: Lowell House, 2000.

Bessel A. van der Kolk, Alexander C. McFarlane, Lars Weisaeth. *Traumatic Stress: The Effects of Overwhelming Experience on Mind, Body, and Society.* New York: The Guilford Press, 2006.

Organizations and Programs

International Critical Incident Stress Foundation, Inc.
3290 Pine Orchard Lane, Suite 106
Ellilcott City, MD 21042
Tel: 410-750-9600
Fax: 410-750-9601
Emergency: 410-313-2473
Website: www.ICISF.org
For information concerning Critical Incident Stress Debriefing Teams and Training.

On-Site Academy

216-222 Mill Street
P.O. Box 1031
Gardner, MA 01440-6031
Tel: 978-632-3518
A Critical Incident Stress Program serving emergency and military personnel from across the nation.

Shalom Retreat and Study Center
664 Cattail Road
Livingston Manor, NY 12758
Tel: 845-482-5421
Contact: Terry Shirreffs
The Art of Loving Retreats (fostering emotional healing and well being).

Al-Anon and ACOA
Tel: 212-870-3400

Alcoholics Anonymous World Service
Tel: 212-870-3400

Narcotics Anonymous
Tel: 818-773-9999

For Veterans assistance contact the local Department of Veteran Affairs Medical Center (VAMC) or Vet Center in your area.

VA Suicide Hotline
Tel: 1-800-273-8255
The toll free hot line connects to the National Suicide Prevention Life-line. Trained personnel from the Department of Veterans Affairs will answer after the #1 is selected.

Healing Books from Resurrection Press

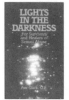

LIGHTS IN THE DARKNESS
For Survivors and Healers of Sexual Abuse

Ave Clark, O.P.

"In her work with survivors and healers, Ave Clark has become a guiding star." —*Gloria Durka*

RP 140/04 ISBN 978-1-878718-12-9   **$8.95**

A PATH TO HOPE
For Parents of Aborted Children and Those Who Minister to Them

John J. Dillon

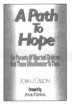

"A 'must' for those who counsel or journey with abortion's second victims." —*The Priest*

RP 020/04 ISBN 978-1-878718-00-6   **$6.95**

HEALING THE WOUNDS OF EMOTIONAL ABUSE
The Journey Worth the Risk

Nancy Benvenga

". . . offers readers both sound principles of guidance and hope-filled resources for prayer and healing." —*Spiritual Book News*

RP 580/04 ISBN 978-1-878718-30-3   **$6.95**

MEDITATIONS FOR SURVIVORS OF SUICIDE
Joni Woelfel

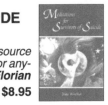

". . . an accessible and truly comforting book. . . . inspiring resource for anyone surviving the suicide of a loved one, or indeed for anyone who grieves." —*Amy Florian*

RP 170/04 ISBN 978-1-878718-75-4   **$8.95**

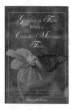

GROWING IN FAITH WHEN
A CATHOLIC MARRIAGE FAILS
For Divorced or Separated Catholics and Those Who Minister with Them

Antoinette Bosco

A source of hope, encouragement and support for divorced Catholics and a healing resource for those who minister in the Catholic community.

RP 748/04 ISBN 978-1-933066-04-2   **$8.95**

THE DILEMMA OF DIVORCED CATHOLICS
Where Do You Stand with the Church?

John T. Catoir, JCD

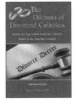

"Father Catoir gives a complete and clear pastoral explanation of both annulments and the 'interior forum' of conscience, with Christ-patterned empathy." —*Antoinette Bosco*

RP 751/04 ISBN 978-1-933066-06-6   **$8.95**

Healing Books from Resurrection Press

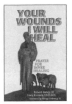

YOUR WOUNDS I WILL HEAL
Prayer for Inner Healing
Robert Faricy, S.J. & Sr. Lucy Rooney, S.N.D.deN.

". . . This book will bring enlightenment and great encouragement to all seeking healing from the Triune God."
—*George A. Maloney, S.J.*

RP 118/04   ISBN 978-1-878718-53-2   **$8.95**

THE HEALING ROSARY
Rosary Meditations for Those in Recovery from Alcoholism and Addictions
Mike D.

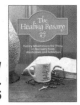

". . . helps us to reappropriate an ancient gift in a very good and needed way."   —*Richard Rohr, O.F.M.*

RP 102/04   ISBN 978-1-878718-40-2   **$5.95**

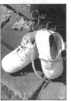

AND A CHILD WILL LEAD
A Path to Healing
Anita M. Constance, S.C.

". . . This book can help all of us to pray our way to a greater trust in a loving and compassionate God."   —*Kathleen Finley*

RP 186/04   ISBN 978-1-878718-88-4   **$7.95**

A RACHEL ROSARY
Intercessory Prayer for Victims of Post-Abortion Syndrome
Larry Kupferman

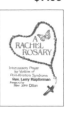

"I can think of no better source of healing for those who are victims of abortion than the intercession of Our Blessed Mother."
—*Msgr. John G. Woolsey*

RP 420/04   ISBN 978-1-878718-21-1   **$4.50**

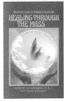

HEALING THROUGH THE MASS
Robert DeGrandis

". . . this fine book will be of great help to you and your loved ones."   —*Bishop Paul V. Dudley*

RP 090/04   ISBN 978-1-878718-10-5   **$8.95**

LESSONS FOR LIVING FROM THE 23RD PSALM
Victor M. Parachin

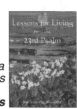

"Each power-packed chapter deconstructs a phrase, offering a heartfelt exploration of its true meaning from someone's life as evidence. . . . This is one to revisit again and again."
—*Crux of the News*

RP 130/04   ISBN 978-1-878718-91-4   **$6.95**

Healing Books from Resurrection Press

Titles by Adolfo Quezada

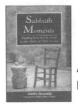

SABBATH MOMENTS
Finding Rest for the Soul in the Midst of Daily Living

A six-week prayer format using Scripture, reflection and prayer.

RP 178/04   ISBN 978-1-878718-80-8   **$6.95**

LOVING YOURSELF FOR GOD'S SAKE

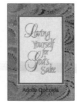

Presents a spirituality of self-love not based on narcissism, but as a response to the divine invitation to self-nurturing.

RP 720/04   ISBN 978-1-878718-35-8   **$5.95**

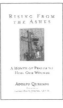

RISING FROM THE ASHES
A Month of Prayer to Heal Our Wounds

". . . helps the reader to heal spiritually and to ask God to give us hope in our present crisis."   **—Fr. Brian Jordan, OFM**

RP 158/04   ISBN 978-1-878718-72-3   **$1.95**

HEART PEACE
Embracing Life's Adversities

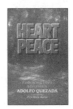

"This is one of the most authentic books I have ever read on the gut wrenching conditions that cause or lead to human suffering. . . . His book is a gift, allowing others to be the beneficiaries of his spiritual journey."   **—Antoinette Bosco**

RP 117/04   ISBN 978-1-878718-52-5   **$9.95**

Titles by Joni Woelfel

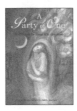

A PARTY OF ONE
Meditations for Those Who Live Alone

This book will comfort and empower those living alone to take ownership for their life, confident in being guided and upheld by God.

RP 744/04   ISBN 978-1-933066-01-1   **$5.95**

THE EDGE OF GREATNESS
Empowering Meditations for Life

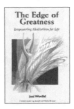

"Here is a woman whose courageous and passionate spirit has enabled her to step over the edge of greatness. Read this book and be blessed."   **—Macrina Wiederkehr, OSB**

RP 134/04   ISBN 978-1-878718-93-8   **$9.95**

Healing Books from Resurrection Press

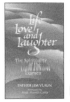

THE SPIRITUAL SPA
Getting Away without Going Away
Mary Sherry

"Perfect for a spiritual centering and an easy read, the book's chapters each end with reflection questions to help you make the most out of the exercises." —*Crux of the News*

RP 745/04   ISBN 978-1-878718-99-0   **$9.95**

BEATITUDES, CHRIST AND THE PRACTICE OF YOGA
A Sacred Log on Land and Sea
Fr. Anthony Randazzo and Madelana Ferrara-Mattheis

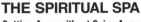

"Embodying the spirit of the Beatitudes through yoga postures can be a means for (re)discovering and renewing our identity as Christians." —*From the Foreword by Fr. Thomas Ryan, CSP*

RP 747/04   ISBN 978-1-933066-00-4   **$9.95**

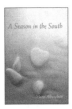

LIFE, LOVE AND LAUGHTER
The Spirituality of the Consciousness Examen
Father Jim Vlaun

" *There is so much simple, shining wisdom in this book."*
—*William J. O'Malley, S.J.*

RP 113/04   ISBN 978-1-878718-43-3   **$7.95**

DISCERNMENT
Seeking God in Every Situation
Rev. Chris Aridas

". . . Aridas provides a practical map for learning how to choose God in our daily lives." —*The Faith Connection*

RP 194/04   ISBN 978-1-878718-88-4   **$8.95**

A SEASON IN THE SOUTH
Marci Alborghetti

". . . honestly portrays the effects of cancer not only on the individual diagnosed but on those that love and care for that person. . . . a treasure for readers everywhere." —*Stephanie Thatcher*

RP 176/04   ISBN 978-1-878718-78-5   **$10.95**

PRAYING THROUGH OUR LIFETRAPS
A Psycho-Spiritual Path to Freedom
John J. Cecero, S.J.

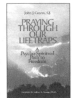

". . . a primer on lifetrap therapy and practice. . . a spiritual guide to finding God in all things." —*Joseph R. Novello, M.D.*

RP 164/04   ISBN 978-1-878718-70-9   **$9.95**

Additional Titles Published by Resurrection Press, a Catholic Book Publishing Imprint

For a free catalog call 1-800-892-6657
www.catholicbookpublishing.com